When
Chicken Soup
Isn't Enough

A VOLUME IN THE SERIES

The Culture and Politics of Health Care Work

Edited by Suzanne Gordon *and* Sioban Nelson

A list of titles in this series is available at www.cornellpress.cornell.edu.

WHEN CHICKEN SOUP ISN'T ENOUGH

Stories of Nurses Standing Up for Themselves, Their Patients, and Their Profession

EDITED BY

SUZANNE GORDON

ILR Press
an imprint of
Cornell University Press
ITHACA AND LONDON

Library of Congress Cataloging-in-Publication Data

When chicken soup isn't enough : stories of nurses standing up for
themselves, their patients, and their profession / edited by Suzanne
Gordon.
    p.   cm.—(The culture and politics of health care work)
   ISBN 978-0-8014-4894-2 (cloth : alk. paper)
   ISBN 978-0-8014-7750-8 (pbk. : alk. paper)
   1. Nursing.   2. Nursing—Social aspects.   3. Communication in nursing.
4. Patient advocacy.   I. Gordon, Suzanne, 1945–   II. Title.   III. Series:
Culture and politics of health care work.
   RT82.W44   2010
   610.73–dc22.   2009051881

Contents

Acknowledgments

I want to thank all the contributors of this book for working so diligently to describe their experiences. I give special thanks to Janine Slome of the South African Forum for Professional Nurse Leaders, Charlotte Thompson of the New Zealand Nurses Organization, David Hughes of the Irish Nurses Organization, Herdis Svensdottir of the University of Iceland School of Nursing, Cecilia Sironi of Varese Hospital and the University of Insubria, Italy, and Amy Garcia at the National Association of Student Nurses (USA) for their help connecting me with some of the contributors to this book. I also thank Ange Romeo-Hall for her stellar editorial work. Emily Zoss also provided critical assistance in shepherding such a large group of authors. My gratitude goes as well to Fran Benson and Sioban Nelson for their support. Finally, I would like to express my appreciation to the amazing editorial, production, and marketing team at Cornell University Press for giving me their encouragement when this idea was in its gestational phase and helping bring it to fruition. Birthing a book, like raising a child, involves a village of people, and thank you to the very best.

Introduction

I've been thinking about putting this book together for several years. During two decades of writing about nursing, I've read many inspirational books, articles, and essays that offer up the literary equivalent of comfort food for RNs. The authors invariably mean to be helpful to the nursing profession by lifting the spirits of its practitioners at a time when so many are feeling tired, stressed out, dispirited, or unappreciated. The problem is, in this heavily sentimental genre, the real-world context of long hours, increased patient loads, and chronic understaffing quickly fades into the background. In the foreground we see traditional images of nurses as people (generally women) who "make a difference" through their touch—always gentle—and niceness. Rarely are their abilities or technical knowledge—represented in a true-to-life setting—the subjects of the story.

In the media, both entertainment and news, and in the imaginations of policymakers and health care administrators, nursing is likewise trivialized as mere hand-holding. When, in 2009, the executive producer of the NBC show *Mercy* described why nurses were chosen as the subject of this new prime-time television drama, she explained her belief that, "by focusing on nurses, it seemed like a way to do a more character-based show set in a hospital. Nurses don't really solve cases, they don't diagnose, so the stories can be more emotionally driven rather than science-driven."

No wonder the public clings to this sentimentalized vision of nurses, and texts that are produced to inspire nurses deliver up story after saccharine story that reinforce traditional stereotypes of nursing and women's work. Nurses are plied from every direction with a narrative that depicts them as modern angels endowed with extra-ordinary powers of empathy and compassion—qualities that are never depicted as the products of education or experience on the job. In the mirror that reflects nursing back to nurses, rarely is it shown that nursing requires more than caring, demanding technical, medical, and pharmacological—to mention only a few—mastery. Just as these texts are soothing and reassuring, so too is the nurses' role in the health care system to be soothing and reassuring: nurses hold hands, anguish over or embrace patients and their families, administer back rubs, or conduct late-night vigils. Both they and their patients seem to be downright etherealized. Indeed, in books like *Chicken Soup for the Nurse's Soul*, the critical intervention of RNs is often powered not by their skill but by their personal belief in ghosts, guiding spirits, or the divine.

It is not surprising that when nurses themselves write in these volumes, they too downplay the extent to which their professional judgment and experience are responsible for positive outcomes. With typical modesty, they minimize the role of RNs in the health care team, at times portraying the nurse as doing little more than being present. These writings thus embrace the notion that professionalism in nursing is an advanced form of self-abnegation. In them female nurses—and male ones, too—are all sugar and spice and everything nice.

Also missing from these well-meaning attempts to honor and celebrate nurses is any mention of the obstacles that many RNs face—and must overcome on a daily basis—as they try to do their jobs well. In the idealized world of these comfort food volumes, there aren't many nurses advocating for patients in the tough, persistent, creative, and courageous manner that I've seen repeatedly in hospitals throughout North America and the world. Typically, these books refer to workplace challenges and issues but gloss right over the crucial tools needed to deal with them: bureaucratic maneuvering, accessing of resources, negotiating with doctors and hospital administrators, and conflict resolution. Nor is there mention of any role for nurses in public policy debates related to health care, or even unity and support among nurses. And what about the contributions made by nursing researchers and teachers in developing new forms of practice or raising the profile of nursing in academic circles? For the nurses in the inspirational narrative, advocacy is a matter of feeling rather than action, having good thoughts but not taking the kinds of personal and professional risks nurses face every day at work as well as in the educational, social, and political arena.

So, as I read this growing body of fundamentally flawed, so-called uplifting literature, I became more convinced that nurses and the public are long overdue for an antidote to the platitudes that purport to feed the nurse's soul. There are so many better stories to tell. We need a collection, I felt, that spotlights the real experience of nurses and their advocacy—in the voices of RNs themselves. Most RNs are simultaneously deeply committed caregivers and advocates willing to stand up for their patients and profession. That's because the best nurses are constantly asserting themselves, in myriad ways, directly and indirectly. They do this as individuals—on their own in conversations with a doctor, a manager, another nurse who is unsupportive, a hospital CEO, COO, or CFO, a journalist or a politician or policymaker, to name only a few. And they do this collectively, as members of professional organizations and unions that are struggling to uphold nursing standards, improve employment conditions, and fight for a better health care system in the United States and around the world.

In the summer of 2008, I went to lunch with some friends who became the focus group for bringing this book to life. They included a professor of nursing, two RN union presidents from the United States, a visiting representative of the Irish Nurses Organization, and a labor relations researcher from Australia.

We all agreed that self-help books of the comfort food variety really aren't helpful at all. To the extent that some nurses are still being socialized—in school and on the job—in the old ways of deference, docility, and self-effacement, these books reinforce outdated notions about how nurses should think and behave. It was time, everyone said, to counter such platitudinous and self-defeating praise for a nursing practice shrouded in self-deprecation. Instead, why not show how nurses break the code of silence and deference every day? Why not spread the word about all those feisty nurses who are the real heroines and heroes in the profession? This conversation fortified my commitment to produce a volume that moved beyond the inspirational to the motivational.

Since that lively lunch meeting, I've gone looking for stories and collected them from dozens of RNs. Nursing groups of all types have put out the call for additional contributors, and many of their members have responded. My goal, from the start, was to have this volume be truly ecumenical as well as international. I wanted to include the first-person accounts of nurses from as many countries as possible. What you find here is the result: stories from nurses from the United States, Canada, England, Australia, New Zealand, Japan, Scandinavia, Iceland, Switzerland, Italy, Ireland, Spain, and more. In this volume you will also hear from nurses in many different institutional roles and settings: bedside nurses and their managers; chief nursing officers; hospice, home care, and school nurses; nurse practitioners and professors; nursing researchers; and organizational leaders. I have divided the book into nine thematic sections, each with a brief introduction, although many of the stories have overlapping motifs.

Because I have asked nurses in a variety of roles to recount their experiences, there are multiple perspectives represented in these pages. The RNs in this book don't necessarily agree with one another. In fact, many disagree passionately about certain issues—such as staffing ratios or unionization for nurses. Some of the stories involve deftly navigated challenges to conventional wisdom, small victories over bureaucratic inertia, or individual acts of resistance to the often-dysfunctional medical domination of our hospital system. Some contributions provide inspiring examples of collective action or health care–related political activity. Some recount how a single nurse stood up for—or to—a patient (e.g., when faced with the threat of physical abuse). Some stories describe complicated interactions with doctors. Some describe tensions among working RNs or between RNs and their managers. Some sections of the book involve people near the top of the health care hierarchy, for example, a nurse executive helping a hospital CEO and board of trustees to do the right thing for patients and his or her profession.

Most of the stories have happy endings. The nurse was able to ensure quality patient care, protect herself or her patient from harm, and successfully advocate or innovate. In some instances, at least in the short term, the nurse was unable to affect needed change but struggled nonetheless. These instances of persistence and courage also provide important lessons. All of the stories offer nurses an alternative to the kind of role model presented in the comfort food literature.

What all of these stories illustrate is the true meaning of advocacy. *Advocacy* is one of the most prominent buzzwords in contemporary nursing. In school, nurses are taught that they must be the patient's advocate. Nurses, as individuals, thus declare proudly that they are patient advocates. Professionally, boards of nursing, nursing organizations, and nurses' codes of ethics proclaim that one of the major roles of the nurse is to advocate for the patient. Like so many words that are used almost reflexively, when nurses say they are patient advocates, or when organizations insist that nurses must advocate for patients, it's not at all clear what they mean by advocacy. Over the years, I've heard nurses loudly trumpet their "advocate" role and then in the next breath tell me they couldn't possibly buck a doctor, a manager, an administrator, speak to a journalist or politician, go on a march or rally, speak out on a controversial issue because their job, promotion, relationships with a pharmaceutical company, professional contacts, or tenure might be at risk. At the height of the restructuring of the 1990s, I remember talking to one chief nurse in Boston about another nurse who'd just lost her job. She was too "pro-nursing" for her own good, he told me. You know, if you stick your neck out like that, well, it's not surprising it gets chopped off. He had no intention of doing that. Of course, I thought, if more managers stuck their necks out, maybe no one's would get chopped off.

I often talk to nurses about telling their stories, revealing inconvenient truths—the kind they tell me about behind closed doors. The kind they say are harming, sometimes even killing their patients. When we then discuss ways to raise these issues, some are terrified. Too terrified to even speak off the record, not for attribution, or even on background. Unlike doctors and many others, nurses don't leak to the media.

Yet, these same nurses still cling to the notion that they are "patient advocates." So, if that is the case, what does *advocacy* mean? I think to some nurses, it means that they want the best for their patients; they wish them well; they hope no harm will come to them. It's a state of mind not a state of action. But advocacy involves—no, demands— action. The very term heralds it. To advocate comes from the Latin word *vocare*—to call. According to Merriam-Webster's dictionary, an *advocate* is one who pleads a cause in a court of law or who defends, vindicates, or espouses a cause by means of argument. Voice is a non-negotiable prerequisite of advocacy. You cannot, after all, "call" out in silence (unless that silence is a silent vigil). It suggests some sort of public speech or action, and it implies the willingness to take risks.

The nurses in this book, like so many millions around the world, have embraced the true meaning of advocacy. Their stories illustrate what it really means to advocate. These stories also extend the meaning of advocacy beyond the traditional role of patient advocate and connect patient advocacy to the act of advocating for nurses' own individual self-respect, well-being, and professionalism.

Whatever their position in the hierarchy or position on controversial nursing and health care issues, the contributors to this book know that they must act and advocate because platitudes are not nourishment enough in our health care system today. They know that to make hospitals and health care institutions a better place for everyone, we need truth telling, more calls to action, and fewer celebrations of a saccharine status quo. In other words, to really feed their souls, nurses know that they need to fight for them.

When
Chicken Soup
Isn't Enough

Part 1
SET UP TO LOSE,
BUT PLAYING TO WIN

For more than two decades, I've had a front-row seat on nurses' socialization in self-denial. Whether in nursing school or on the job, nurses are taught how to care for and be concerned about patients. They are constantly enjoined to advocate for patients. What they are not encouraged to do is to advocate for, or even acknowledge, their own needs either as human beings or as professionals. Sometimes I think nurses are taught that altruism means they have no needs at all.

I watched this play out in the early 1990s when I was writing about nursing at the Beth Israel Hospital in Boston for my book *Life Support: Three Nurses on the Front Lines*. I spent several years following nurses at the Hematology-Oncology Outpatient Clinic. They were amazing and delivered exquisite patient care. What they had trouble with was sticking up for themselves. The nurses worked with patients whose outcomes were grim. Over 50 percent died. The work took an emotional toll. The institution recognized this, and every few weeks, it offered what were called psych rounds. A psychiatric nurse came to facilitate a discussion about their work. Ostensibly they could freely air their concerns, frustration, sadness, even their despair.

Problem was, they didn't feel the psychiatric nurse was helpful. Even more inhibiting, their manager insisted on being present during these meetings. They wanted a new facilitator (they had a person who was willing to do the job), and they didn't want their manager present. After each meeting they would complain among themselves about the facilitator and about the fact that their manager's presence inhibited their ability to comfortably express their concerns.

1

For two years, these nurses vented their frustration after each session and vowed to do something to change things the next. They never did. They simply didn't know how to prepare their case, work together for themselves, and make their argument.

Of course, no matter where we work, we all face the choice of do I speak up or remain silent? And, if I take a stand, what should the issue be? But these nurses seemed to be fighting with their hands tied behind their backs. They weren't supposed to have needs, or if they had them, they were supposed to sacrifice them for the good of the patient or their institution or their profession. They had not learned what I had learned in the women's movement and from the struggles of other oppressed groups—that is, how to network, strategize, and organize to get what you have long deserved. I wanted to intervene, to advise, to suggest ideas, but I was there as a journalistic observer not as a workplace adviser. Because I kept quiet when I knew I could have helped, it made me feel almost as frustrated as they did.

That's why I begin with the stories in this first section. Here, we have nurses from every corner of the profession as well as from around the globe who have advocated for what they need and won. They questioned physician decisions that jeopardized patient care and challenged the reorganization schemes of hospital consultants who know far less about nursing than veteran RNs and nurse managers. They refused to accept workplace behavior that was improper and sometimes even illegal. As individuals and collectively, they challenged conventional wisdom that stood in the way of much-needed change for themselves, their patients, and coworkers. And, for them, winning felt really good!

A Covert Operation

Kathleen Bartholomew

I was a brand new manager with absolutely no experience, but I knew intuitively that to run the fifty-seven bed orthopedic and spine units effectively, I would have to cultivate a relationship with their physicians. The orthopedic physicians met every Friday morning at seven for rounds where two physicians would present their most difficult cases. While the first and second physicians were switching out x-rays, I asked if I could talk to the doctors to establish a definite time and place for weekly communication. Thereafter, every week at "half-time" (i.e., halfway through rounds), I would get five precious minutes to speak to the orthopedic doctors. This time was invaluable. It allowed me to address unit problems, relay critical trends in care, and bring the concerns of nursing to our physician partners.

The spine doctors were a different story. Month after month I would ask them to meet, and no one would show up. I was frustrated. How could I get the neuro and ortho doctors on the same page if I couldn't even talk to them? This was a new unit, and there was a lot of work to be done. One day, one of the spine physicians stopped by my office, and I asked him point blank why the attendance at my meetings was slim to none.

"Because we already meet once a month at a physician's house," he replied. "It's called 'Journal Club,' and we are meeting tomorrow night. . . . So no one is going to go to your meeting today when we can all see each other tomorrow evening."

"Whose house are you meeting at?" I replied curiously.

"Why, Doctor Wagner's," he replied slowly.

"Great," I said boldly, "I'll need directions." Reluctantly, he gave me the address.

The next evening I drove through one of the most expensive areas in all of Seattle until I pulled up in front of a huge mansion on the water. Nervously, I approached the front door. My heart was beating so loudly that you could have taken my pulse by just looking at me. The giant door-knocker reminded me of the scene from *The Wizard of Oz* where Dorothy is shaking uncontrollably as the wizard's voice booms. But as I approached the door, I saw a small note posted there that read, "Just come right on in."

AGH! It was difficult enough to knock on the door, but to *"just walk in?"* Nervously I opened the huge solid oak door and followed the trail of voices through the massive entry hall into a dining room clearly intended for a king. The view of the lake was breathtaking. As I came around the corner, I could see three spine physicians eating pizza and drinking beer while waiting for the rest of the group to arrive. The room reeked of testosterone. For just an instant, shock and disbelief flashed across their faces, escaping only briefly before being politely recalled. Suddenly, I felt like a covert operator infiltrating enemy ranks.

Graciously, the physicians offered me a drink and I sat down at the table. When the entire group arrived, one by one, they shared their assignments, which were reviews of the latest journal articles, as I sat silently without ever saying a word. Clearly, this was not the time or place for a discussion on the problems the nurses were having on the unit with the various physician orders. I sat and listened through the evening.

Even though it was a struggle at times to follow some of their complicated jargon, I came the next three months as well. Finally, after the fourth month, a physician said, "Kathleen, why don't you present next week?"

"I would love to," I replied. "The nurses have noticed that some physician's patients are up walking faster than others and we have linked that to the use of Toradol post-op. I would like to present the research on this topic."

I can think of nothing that elevated the profession of nursing more in the eyes of those physicians than the nursing research I presented at these meetings for a year. At last, we felt like we were at the same table. The nurses joked and said that I belonged at Journal Club because I had "the balls to even go in the first place." The change was gradual, but over the months my relationships with the spine physicians became more comfortable, and I no longer shook with fear as I approached their houses. Physicians gave me more of their time on the unit where I did bring up the problems with various order sets, and we eventually reviewed these at a Journal Club meeting. I called them by their first names, just as they called me by mine. Finally, despite the differences in education, class, role, and gender, it felt like we were actually partners in patient care—thanks to a successful covert mission.

· · ·

KATHLEEN BARTHOLOMEW, RN, RC, MN, is a Practicing Orthopedic Nurse and national nursing speaker, as well as author of *Ending Nurse to Nurse Hostility, Speak Your Truth: Strategies to Improve RN/MD Relationships, Stressed Out about Communication*, and coauthor of *Our Image, Our Choice*.

Saving Patients from Dr. Death

Toni Hoffman

I first met the surgeon who came to be known as "Dr. Death" when he was hired to work in our small rural hospital, Bundaberg Base Hospital, in Southeast Queensland in 2003, where I was nurse unit manager in the intensive care unit. Dr. Jayant Patel, who's been implicated in eighty-seven patient deaths and was hired as a general surgeon, came to us from the United States. No one had ever really checked up on him—and no one had ever bothered even to Google him. That would have saved a lot of lives and a lot of anguish.

Only three weeks after his arrival, Dr. Patel was promoted to director of surgery. It didn't take much longer to recognize that there were problems with his behavior and competence. Almost straightaway, he began to sexually harass staff. For example, while examining a sick patient in the ICU, he asked a female staff member for her phone number and then repeatedly called her at home to ask her out. He also wanted to perform the types of surgery that were way beyond the kind usually performed in our small hospital and had been—before his arrival—routinely transferred to larger hospitals in Brisbane. Although I and other nurses were very concerned about Dr. Patel, he quickly built up a strong rapport with our chief executive. He would say that he could do whatever he wanted because he was earning so much money for the hospital.

I lodged my first complaint about Dr. Patel five weeks after his arrival. His patients were coming to the ICU with serious complications—for example, with wounds—that we had not seen before. Operating theater staff would say, "Oh, Dr. Patel has nicked a liver or spleen," but these incidents were never documented. Nothing happened when I lodged my complaint, and problems like these went on. I tried to approach other colleagues, but no one would do anything. I put in another complaint in June 2004, after a patient

6

who'd suffered a serious chest injury wasn't transferred quickly enough to Brisbane and died. Dr. Patel had interfered with the transfer.

I made my complaint, and the administration turned against me. The director of nursing, the district manager (hospital CEO), and the director of medical services claimed that this was a personality conflict and that I had trouble with conflict resolution skills. They also labeled me a racist. The focus had clearly shifted from him to me.

Nonetheless, the nurses in the ICU were trying to stop Dr. Patel from operating on patients. The medical doctors were, by that time, aware of the problems. Behind his back they were calling him "Dr. Death" and saying things like, "If I come in here, don't let him near me." Some did complain about him, but when they went to the executive, they were ignored. So we would conspire with the doctors to transfer patients out to Brisbane before Patel could get to them. Toward the end we were actually hiding patients from Patel.

After I put in my big complaint, the executive gave Patel an employee of the month award. That made it crystal clear that our complaints were not and would not be acted on. I spoke with other agencies within Queensland Health. I spoke to the coroner, the police, and the nurses' union. Toward the end, I decided I had to go outside the organization. So I went to see a member of Parliament, Rob Messenger—who was in the opposition National Liberal Party. (Queensland had a Labour Party government.) I also contacted a journalist named Hedley Thomas.

At first Messenger didn't believe me either. He rang up a doctor in town who said, "Yes, we know about Dr. Patel, and we hope he will go away quietly." Dr. Patel's visa was soon to expire. But finally, Messenger presented my letter of complaint in the Queensland Parliament.

Shortly after, Hedley Thomas came to our hospital to talk to the nurses. Then he did what no one else had ever done. He Googled Patel and discovered that his problematic history dated all the way back to 1981. He had been first disciplined for falsifying records and relinquished his license to practice in 2001 rather than face prosecution. He also had the dubious honor of being the most sued surgeon at Kaiser Permanente in Portland, Oregon. He wasn't allowed to perform surgery in the United States. Then, of course, all hell broke loose, and the story emerged in public.

Patel fled back to Portland, Oregon, but was extradited in July of 2008. He is out on bail, awaiting trial on three manslaughter charges, several grievous bodily harm charges, and fraud. Because the Labour Party was in government and I went to a National Party member, there were significant political ramifications. The health minister was fired and was just sentenced to seven years in jail on corruption charges. The director general for health lost his job. Not to mention the poor patients who suffered or died. Dr. Patel operated on 1,400 people in the two years he was here and has been involved in at least eighty-seven deaths. But no one really knows how many people he harmed or killed.

For me, standing up for my patients was a difficult experience. Some people supported me and some didn't. A lot of people can't forgive me for going outside the institution. But I had to do it. And if the same thing happened again, I would do it all over. I hope, because of our efforts to stop Dr. Patel, I will never have to.

· · ·

TONI HOFFMAN, AM, BN, Graduate Certificate in Management, Master of Bioethics, is the Nurse Unit Manager in ICU at Bundaberg Base Hospital, Bundaberg, Queensland, Australia.

A Lesson for the Principal

Kathy Hubka

School nurses take care of kids with increasingly serious health issues. Kids with asthma, diabetes, and epilepsy. To do our jobs, we give out meds. People know pills go down people's throats, but they are often unaware of the other orifices through which medications are delivered. That was certainly the case with a principal in one of the schools I coordinated in Wichita, Kansas.

Because I was a coordinator of school nurses for the school system, principals would give me a heads up if they were planning to cut staff. So I wasn't surprised to get a call from a principal informing me that he planned to decrease the amount of time the school nurse would be at the school. To make sure that would be safe, I asked him about the needs of the kids in his school. Did any have asthma? Yes, he answered.

Well, I said, a non-nurse could be delegated to deal with inhalers.

What about other health problems? I asked. Did any of the students have epilepsy and if so, did they take Diastat (i.e., a rectal form of valium). Well, guess what? It turned out that one did. I asked him if he knew how that medication was administered? He said he wasn't too sure. I explained that it was a medication that could be delegated to a non-nurse but is given rectally. He let out a gasp and asked, "Well, who would do that?"

I answered, based on my prior experience working in schools, "The medicine could be delegated to you and you could be called upon to give it in case of emergency."

Another gasp and then silence.

That's when he started to think, "Well, maybe I can find funding to keep the nurse."

And he did.

· · ·

KATHY HUBKA, RN, BSN, NCSN, is Coordinator of Health Services, Wichita Public Schools.

The Delicate Discharge

Ruth Johnson

As Robert Frost once observed, home is the place where, when you have to go there, they have to take you in. Mr. Smith's "medical home" is our emergency room, where he gets dropped off every few months by the police or the EMTs, depending on whether he has attacked someone or has been attacked. He usually comes in screaming and cursing at everyone in sight. Once here, he tells us all about his powerful suicidal urges and how his prescription medications ran out and he has been forced to resort to a combination of street drugs again. He hasn't held a job in years and is usually homeless. And we take him in.

When he arrives on our locked psychiatric unit, Mr. Smith's behavior changes. Because he has a history of assaulting others, he rates a private room in our Intensive Psychiatric Care area. This includes an en suite bathroom, cable television, and as much food as he can eat. After a hot meal and a shower, Mr. Smith becomes quiet and refined. He occasionally joins other patients to watch a movie or sports event, but otherwise he stays in his room and keeps to himself. He declines— with varying degrees of profanity—to participate in any of our therapeutic groups or other treatment modalities and will only engage in conversations about his medication dosages.

But Mr. Smith reverts to his "911" behavior during morning rounds. When the doctors inquire about his thoughts and feelings, he insists that he is still suicidal, with several sure-fire plans to do himself in, and he expresses great fear that he would be unable to keep himself safe outside the hospital. When the social worker raises the question of discharge planning, Mr. Smith raises his voice to declare that a discharge order would be his death warrant. He has been known to rant at some length on the subject, and once in a while he throws things. When rounds end, Mr. Smith returns calmly to his room and calls for his medication.

Unfortunately for Mr. Smith, his government insurance eventually determines that he no longer meets criteria for hospital level of care. The insurance company has its standards and routines, and we at our hospital unit have ours. When we learn that a patient is to be unwillingly discharged, we get our ducks in a row to make it a safe and efficient process.

Unfortunately for the staff and patients on our unit, Mr. Smith's day of discharge was the first day of our new resident psychiatrist's tour of duty. Our young Dr. Kildare was a congenial woman who cheerfully shared pictures of her children with the nurses and took notes as we filled her in on each of her patients. She and I agreed that this was to be Mr. Smith's day of departure. But then our beepers called us in different directions, and the next time I saw her she was, to my deep horror, standing in Mr. Smith's doorway and telling him that he would be discharged this very day. From the hallway I could hear him shouting "You can't discharge me! I'm suicidal! I have my rights! You're signing my death warrant!" Thumping sounds came from inside his room. Dr. Kildare retreated into the hallway and looked a bit startled.

"I seem to have agitated him a bit," she confided to me. "Let me know if you need an order for a PRN med or something." Her beeper squawked and she was gone.

The horses were out of the barn now, and everyone on the hallway could hear them kicking. Our motto is "safety first," so I called for security backup and then went to Mr. Smith's doorway. He was in "911" mode, but underneath it all I knew that he truly believed in the healing power of drugs.

"Ahhh, Mr. Smith, can I get you a PRN with your morning meds?"

"Sure," he shouted, "anything you got is FINE!" Thump.

A quartet of our largest security officers arrived on the scene, and I went to pour Mr. Smith's meds. He seemed to find the presence of four Men in Black reassuring, and he had stopped swinging at the walls when I returned with an overflowing cup of pharmaceuticals. He took them in one gulp, then sat down on his bed and waited for the magic to happen.

I paged Dr. Kildare. She had been proceeding to round on her other patients. I explained to her that, having told Mr. Smith of his discharge, she needed to drop whatever she was doing and finish his discharge paperwork immediately, for the safety of everyone including our patient.

"Uh, does he need a chemical restraint?" she asked. The word "safety" had registered with her.

"Not yet. That's why you need to get moving on this. If he gets a chemical, he'll be off his feet till tomorrow because we can't send an impaired patient outside. And in the meantime we're tying up four security officers and closing doors all over the unit to keep from scaring the paranoid patients."

"I see. Okay, I'll get right on it." I could hear her beeper squawk as she hung up.

Mr. Smith put on his call light. When I arrived, he had changed into his street clothes and was packing his bag under the benign gaze of Security.

"I have to go right now," he said darkly. "Once I know I'm going, I have to leave right away. Now."

"We're happy to help you with that," I responded, "but we're waiting for the paperwork to be processed. And your social worker needs to set up your outpatient appointments in the computer before she can issue your *cab voucher.*" I emphasized the last because it was something worth waiting for.

"NOW!" he yelled and pushed past me into the hallway. He greased through the Security gauntlet and flung himself against the locked ICU door. He pounded his fists against the shatterproof glass screaming, "You're signing my death warrant! You're all killers!"

The security officers carefully folded Mr. Smith's arms down and toted him back to his room. They resumed chatting with him about last night's playoffs while the entire staff of our unit went on red alert. The hallway between Mr. Smith's room and the locked outside door was cleared of all objects. All traffic on the unit was detoured toward another hallway. Upset patients were talked to and comforted. Some even needed extra medication before they could calm themselves. And nobody thought about going to lunch.

It took an hour for Dr. Kildare to enter the discharge orders, follow-up appointments, and prescriptions into the computer system. She continued to field beeper and phone calls through the process, and she had to do the orders again when I pointed out the typos. When she emerged from her office with the prescriptions and discharge papers in hand, the unit was silent.

Mr. Smith understood that he had negotiated the best possible outcome for himself and could now afford to be generous. He picked up his bag and marched toward the front door, flanked by his security phalanx. He waved to me, calling out, "Thanks for everything, honey." Two sets of locked doors swung wide open for him, then whooshed closed. Our unit exhaled.

My colleagues sent me off for an excellent lunch break, making sure that I took time to savor a hot fudge sundae, followed by some deep breathing. After that I was feeling as expansive as Mr. Smith and decided that this was a Teachable Moment for young Dr. Kildare. I took her aside.

"I know this was stressful for you," she began somewhat defensively, "but I don't see how it could have played out any differently."

"It could and it does," I replied. "We're all one team, and if you come to us, we'll tell you what the plays are. The key here is to talk to the nurses who know him well, which you started to do but then got distracted. We could have told you that he would get dangerously upset. The thing to do is to set up his discharge paperwork *first*, then call Security to set up a time that is good for them. When all of our ducks are in a row, you and I have security behind us when we break the news to the patient. Security gets him dressed and packed and out the door in a matter of minutes. And then we all get lunch on time."

"Oh. You can really do it that way?"

"Sure. Just ask. Your job is hard enough, you might as well play with the home team."

She accepted my offer of a dark chocolate truffle, which was probably her only lunch. Turns out, she has a *very* sharp learning curve.

• • •

RUTH JOHNSON, MSN, MPA, CNM, is an advanced practice psychiatric nurse specializing in women's mental health.

No Patience for Poison

Brenda Carle

My fingers gently lift my patient's swollen eyelids to look into his eyes as he is recovering from coronary artery bypass surgery. I move the small light to assess pupil reaction. As I explain the reasons for my neurological assessment to my nonresponding patient, I'm asking myself, "Why is he not waking up? Surgery was two days ago!"

I smile at his wife who anxiously watches me as I confirm his stable cardiac rhythm, monitor his blood pressure, and ensure the vasoactive medications that are dripping into his central line catheter have not leaked into the skin.

It's the moment for me to question everything: Have we prevented air embolism, deep vein thrombosis, arterial occlusion? Have cerebral perfusion pressures been adequate? Is cardiac output consistently stable? Is he oxygenating well? Consider lab results. Consider medication effect. I want to collaborate with the cardiothoracic surgeon to brainstorm etiology of comatose state post surgery and intervene to improve patient status.

The cardiologist is standing at the chart now and with a quick look into the room casually comments, "Still hasn't woken up yet? Let's give him more time."

As he walks away, I say, "I am curious about his thiocyanate level since he is on nitroprusside to control his hypertension. Or can we get a CT scan to rule out stroke?"

The physician does not turn around and says, "We don't need to get unnecessary tests! His renal function is fine." I could have said "okay" and carried on with my other work, but my education and experience led me to challenge the physician's view. It was my responsibility to ensure a better patient outcome, decrease length of stay and cost, alleviate the patient's suffering and the emotional turmoil of the patient's wife.

14

I hit the phone and called Tucson Poison Control. The official I talked to agreed that a thiocyanate level should be ordered. We got the specimen, and guess what? Its toxicity was leading to my patient's loss of consciousness. Feeling elated that we found a potential reason for my patient's unresponsive state, I called the surgeon to report the toxic level. I heard silence, then his calm reply: "Thank you. Please turn off the nipride and watch the BP." I turned the nitroprusside drip off. My patient woke up within hours.

When the surgeon came to see the patient, the patient was sitting up in bed, with eyes wide open and stable neurological status restored. The surgeon cracked a smile of disbelief and appreciation, and said, "Brenda, thank you," while meeting my eyes.

As a nurse, I felt proud that I questioned the status quo and challenged a colleague for the benefit of safe patient care. I earned the respect of a cardiothoracic surgeon. I received hugs from my patient's wife. Most important, I protected my patient.

· · ·

Brenda Carle, RN, BSN, PCCN, is a Clinical Educator of Progressive Critical Care Unit and Central Monitoring, Tucson Medical Center, Tucson, Arizona.

Mr. CEO, Will You Marry Me?

Candice Owley

For many years, as president of the Wisconsin Federation of Nurses and Health Professionals, I have negotiated collective bargaining contracts for registered nurses. In the vast majority of cases, the bargaining team is predominantly female and the employer's team is overwhelmingly male. This gender disparity has led to many interesting conversations filled with stereotypes of women and nurses. For example, because so many nurses are women, they don't need a raise because they aren't the major breadwinners in the family. Or how about this one: Nurses/women should always have back-up babysitters handy so that they can work forced overtime and don't have to take time off because of a sick child. Fortunately, attitudes such as these have—for the most part—become part of a past culture. Over time, everyone realized that many women are single parents or the major source of household income. Recently, however, when bargaining in a small Midwestern town, I was reminded that old habits die hard.

A group of about one hundred nurses were in contract negotiations with the largest health care employer in the state of Wisconsin. Since these were the only unionized nurses out of over twenty thousand employees in the system, the power difference was immense. Yet the nurses were a feisty bunch who were very willing to fight for their rights. As they began bargaining a replacement contract, they knew they would be facing pension cuts; the twenty thousand non-union workers had already had their pensions reduced. This proposal was shocking since this was in the middle of the most serious nursing shortage the country had faced in decades. One would think that hospitals would be increasing nurses' benefits, not reducing them.

As the chief negotiator and a nurse myself, I made a strong argument to management that they should be increasing not reducing the current, already modest pension benefit. To make our case, I highlighted the fact that women are more apt to end up in poverty in retirement, and so it was even more important to improve pension benefits. Much to my surprise, the hospital's chief negotiator chose to make light of my comments by responding, "if nurses want better pensions they should MARRY WELL."

The nurses were outraged. Even if meant as a joke, we had come too far in our quest for equality to let such a sexist comment go without protest. The nurses responded by putting out a leaflet to the other union members expressing their anger. We expected an apology or retraction at the next bargaining session but instead the hospital representative chastised the local president for making a big deal out of an offhand comment. The battle was on.

The hospital system CEO was extremely well paid, with over $3 million per year in wages and pension benefits. The nurses decided that the CEO was evidently the type of husband the hospital negotiator must have had in mind for them. So the nurses scavenged the local second-hand stores for bridal dresses. We then rented a bus and dozens of middle-aged nurses wearing wedding dresses and nurses' caps with veils attached marched to the CEO's office to "propose" marriage. "Marry Us," the signs they held implored.

The press on the event was fantastic with both local and national coverage. Over forty TV stations reported on the story. Following the tremendously successful press event, the nurses took out newspaper ads, flew an aerial banner over the Fourth of July fireworks display, held a community rally, and mailed a ballot to over thirty thousand area nurses asking whose pension should be cut: nurses' or the CEO's. You can guess how that vote turned out.

Still there was no settlement, so the nurses turned up the heat with billboards, letters to the editor, radio ads, and yard signs delivered by nurse-brides.

After months of battling, the hospital finally agreed to a cash settlement of $250,000 for the nurses to offset the pension cuts. Money that none of the twenty thousand other employees received. As part of the victory celebration, the nurse-brides led the local Labor Day parade riding in a caravan of convertibles. While the nurses would have preferred stopping the pension cuts, they were proud of both their victory and willingness to stand and fight for their rights. They took on the bully and won.

• • •

CANDICE OWLEY, RN, is President of Wisconsin Federation of Nurses and Health Professionals, Chairperson of AFT Healthcare, and an executive board member of Public Services International.

Intolerable Behavior

Eleanor Geldard

I was the unit manager of a multidisciplinary intensive care unit at a private hospital in South Africa. One day, the twelve-bed ICU was full, and it happened to be visiting hours. One of the patients—a multiple gunshot victim—was on a ventilator and, although awake, was quite ill and unstable. His principal doctor, a trauma surgeon, had seen the patient early in the morning and had written numerous orders for the patient. The nurse looking after the patient was a black woman who took immense pride in her work and always gave her patients comprehensive and empathetic care.

The patient's wife and mother were by his side. A small-statured, white cardiothoracic surgeon (Dr. X), also looking after the patient, then entered the room without introducing himself and began reading through the chart. Dr. X was unpopular among hospital staff because of his infamous temper tantrums and abusive behavior. Many nurses in the ICU refused to work with him because of this. A few moments later, Dr. X glanced up from the chart and questioned the nurse as to why things had been changed. She informed him the trauma surgeon had ordered all changes. Dr. X turned red, stamped his feet, slammed his hand on the table, and shouted at the nurse that she had "no right" to change the ventilator and other vitriol such as "You are fucking stupid" and "Where did you train—at a hairdressing salon?"

The nurse remained calm, but I could see she was hurt, embarrassed, and upset. The patient, his family, and, by now, other patients, visitors, and staff on the unit were listening to this unfolding drama. The nurse offered repeatedly to get the trauma surgeon on the phone, so that Dr. X could talk to him about his management of the patient. Dr. X ignored these offers, continuing to shout that the changes were stupid and that we were killing the patient. Then came the cherry on the cake. He screamed at my nurse, "You are a stupid, fucking, black, kaffir bitch." (*Kaffir* is a very derogatory term for a black African.)

I had had enough of his abuse and racism. I walked up to him, grabbed him by his collar and dragged him to the door, pushed him out, told him he was not welcome in my unit, and slammed the door shut. As it was an electronically locked door, he couldn't get back in and stood there hammering and kicking at it and yelling at me.

I immediately went to the patient and family to calm them down and apologized for the doctor's behavior. I apologized to all the patients and visitors—feeling humiliated that they should witness such unprofessional and unnecessary behavior. My nurse was shattered—she was sobbing uncontrollably and said she wanted to leave the profession of nursing. It took twenty minutes to calm her down and convince her to stay. At this point, I received a phone call from the hospital manager—he wanted to see me in his office.

When I walked in, Dr. X was standing there fuming. The hospital manager asked if it was true that I had thrown the surgeon out of ICU. I said yes and told him why. After hearing the details, the hospital manager supported me and informed Dr. X that his behavior would no longer be tolerated. At no stage did the surgeon offer any kind of apology to the patient, family, or any of my staff. About a week later, I happened to be standing in the corridor having a discussion with another doctor when Dr. X walked past. He turned and pulled on my sleeve and asked me, "Are we friends yet?" Apart from the fact that I found his interruption rude, I was also irked at his question and replied, "If you want my friendship doctor, earn it first." He looked at me, somewhat shocked, and simply walked away.

From that point on whenever Dr. X came into our ICU, he behaved well. It's amazing how effective the knowledge was that he would be reported for any future misbehavior in helping him control his temper.

• • •

ELEANOR GELDARD, RN, works in the private health care sector in South Africa.

One Is One Too Many

Thomas Smith

As chief nursing officer (CNO) in a hospital, it is my job to preserve the integrity of my organization's community of nurses—a community that provides the foundation of our ability to serve patients and the wider community. Sometimes doing this is one of the most significant challenges for a CNO.

This was a challenge I constantly faced in the 1990s when consultants were pouring through health care organizations undergoing financial difficulties. One of these firms landed in the hospital whose nursing department I led at the time. The hospital was in deep financial trouble, and the consultants had dozens of metrics to demonstrate how many dollars we needed to cut. They presented me with a proposal to significantly reduce the nursing budget and nurse full-time equivalent positions (FTEs).

I was keenly aware of the urgent need to reduce our financial deficit. Nonetheless, I looked at their proposal and I said no. I told the consultants that I was determined to meet the target and that I was committed to working relentlessly to achieve that goal. But not by laying off nurses.

To no one's surprise, the consultants were skeptical. "There's no way you can achieve this goal without laying off nurses," they responded. "We'll see," I said to myself.

In spite of skepticism from the consultants and some of my peers, I moved ahead. My first step was calling together the senior nursing leadership team. We brainstormed about options that could allow us to reach the financial target without having to resort to RN layoffs.

Working closely with the unions was our next step. I personally met with union leaders to let them know about the dire nature of the current situation and the organization's immediate need to shed expenses. I added that I had some ideas to prevent layoffs, and that I was certain the union would have some as well.

Building on this dialogue and exchange, we identified a number of strategies that would avoid layoffs. We planned to offer nurses the opportunity to take a leave of absence while maintaining their benefits. Such an offer would allow nurses to continue their health insurance and maintain their seniority in the organization, but they would leave the payroll for a certain period of time. This proposal turned out to meet the personal goals of some nurses because it meant they could go to school, take care of family members or concerns, or even plan a long-desired trip.

Another idea was a temporary reduction of work hours, while still allowing the continuation of prereduction benefits. With this approach, benefits such as tuition reimbursement continued, but the trade-off was a cut in weekly payroll expenses. Also planned was an offer of early retirement for those who were eligible.

We modeled all these options and then performed the calculations. If our assumptions were right, and there was staff buy-in, we would be able to meet the financial target.

With the plan now formulated, I communicated it to the entire nursing staff in round-the-clock meetings. In more than twenty-five years as a nurse leader, I have never conducted so many meetings with so many people in the same room. People knew about the crisis, and they poured in. We had handed out all the details of the plan ahead of time and had resolved some points of contention with the union. Nurses understood the seriousness of the crisis and the options that our plan could offer them.

In spite of protests from the consultants who proclaimed that no financial reduction could be implemented without handing out pink slips, I then put the plan into action. The outcome was successful. No one received a single pink slip! We were able to reach the target without laying off even one nurse.

To this day, I feel intensely proud of our achievement. For me, the most satisfying aspect of this experience was the collaborative approach that engaged the entire community of nurses. We certainly understood that the consultants had a charge they needed to fulfill. But we wanted to demonstrate that we could meet the target without damaging the fabric of our culture and our community. We knew that the injury from the subsequent trauma and loss would have taken a long time to heal.

Throughout this process, I remained passionate and firm in my conviction that the integrity of our community of nurses was at stake. Loss of a significant portion of our community would have been a fundamental violation and wound. I knew I had to do everything I could to prevent it. I worked with my colleagues, partners, friends—whomever I could gather in a room—to ensure that wasn't going to happen. To this day, my philosophy remains the same: One layoff is one too many.

· · ·

Thomas Smith, MS, RN, NEA-BC, is Senior Vice President, Nursing and Hospital Operations, Maimonides Medical Center, Brooklyn, New York.

A Comfortable Cover Up

Jenny Kendall

Who cares how someone is dressed while in hospital? I do. If people were dressed in the streets as they are in hospital they would be charged with indecent exposure.

After having spent over three decades in the operating theaters at Wellington Hospital as a second-level nurse, my concern about this issue is long-standing. No one was prepared to listen. That changed in August 2007.

Working as a nurse in New Zealand, I had been observing unease and discomfort of patients of all ages, especially among Maori and Pacific Island people coming to operating theater for surgery. They'd been given only an open-backed nightie and "one size fits all" pants— which often don't get worn. Alternately, they would come in their own clothes and be asked to change into a nightie before going into theater.

As Maori and Pacific Islanders traditionally have their legs covered, I strongly believe it is culturally insensitive for us, as providers, not to offer more appropriate attire to vulnerable patients while in hospital. This led me to believe that we were not providing a safe environment for patients.

I embarked on a journey to improve the situation. Over the past decade, I had visited the Pacific Islands on a regular basis, and I had noticed that patients in the operating theaters there wear a *lava-lava*—a wrap-around bottom—and a top. This gave me the idea of introducing something similar in New Zealand.

I made an appointment with the theater manager and discussed my concerns. She gave me the green light to deal with the problem, which included accessing the data on the ethnicity of patients coming to the operating theater for any procedure. Now I had the freedom, if not the time, to do this project, which was an addition to my full-time schedule and rotating hours.

This journey was not the smoothest. In addition to the time factor, nurses who didn't want to change presented a second challenge. My strategy? To win over these nurses, I needed to demonstrate that I had the support from the group manager for theaters to take on this project and see it through.

My journey started with meetings with the management of both the Pacific Island Support Unit and the Maori Health Unit, and regular attendance at the South Pacific Nurses Forum, which gave me confidence to go and talk to community groups and hospital workers from other ethnicities. To validate my concerns, I had to process two years' worth of data. I wanted to know the percentage of patients coming to the operating theaters who were of ethnicities that traditionally had their legs covered. The results proved my concerns were legitimate; 29 percent of patients fell into this category.

Having demonstrated the need for change with the data, we conducted an informal trial within the theater suite, with all patients having a blanket folded around them after surgery. No more exposure when turning on their sides in the Post Anesthesia Care Unit. Our plan was to start here and have all of the wards in the hospital adopt the modified garment.

After two monthly meetings with nursing management were deferred, I rang the wards myself and made an appointment on my days off to go and talk to the staff and show them how to use the garment. I called a meeting with theater management, the Maori Health Unit, and the Pacific Island Support Unit, and we agreed on a process to try out the garment in some of the surgical wards. We had to get the buy-in from the laundry service that would be laundering and dispatching the garment throughout the hospitals. Suitable material was purchased and put through rigorous testing in the laundry and given the green light.

I went to the selected wards and spoke to the charge nurse manager, explaining what the trial was about and asking if they were interested in participating. They all agreed to assist with the trial and ask the patients to fill in an evaluation form before they left the hospital.

A formal trial was launched for a period of three months. Surgical patients were offered the use of a blanket to wear to theater and back to the ward. Along with the blankets, we provided Pacific Island–styled *lava lavas* as an option.

At the launch, the New Zealand Minister of Pacific Island Affairs acknowledged the initiative as something that was a concern and was pleased that I had chosen to remedy it. We received a Certificate of Appreciation from the New Zealand Human Rights Commission's Race Relation Commissioner because the project included all ethnicities and nationalities.

With no formal computer training in conducting research, certainly not with spreadsheets and graphs, I had to learn fast. One of my nursing colleagues came to the rescue and within a week I had sufficient knowledge to get on with processing the data I had collected. I spent long evenings in the medical library or after hours at work using the computers. Of the ninety-nine responses from patients during the three-month trial period, 85 percent supported using a garment to cover the midsection of patients.

During the trial, other wards and departments asked if they could use the garment. I gained permission to do a six-week audit of all patients arriving in theater. I asked them whether they would be interested in wearing such a garment. The response was overwhelmingly positive. In fact, 60 percent of people identifying themselves as European wanted to wear it. Some 597 responses were received, and 90 percent were in favor of being given the option of wearing a wraparound garment while in hospital.

While this initiative started off in the operating theaters, word got around and it quickly was extended to the wards. This helped make it easier to support the purchasing of specially made garments.

The official launch for the implementation was held on September 22, 2008. Members of Parliament, diplomats, government officials, and members of community groups attended. We received a lot of media attention for both the trial and the implementation of this initiative. The laundry services management came on board with the offer to purchase the garments and carry them as a stock item that can be ordered along with other linen.

The garments have been well received, and some nurses are finding that patients using them have become more independent and are up and about more quickly. People from all ethnicities are wearing them, and there is a big demand for them in the clinics.

This initiative is a first for any hospital in New Zealand, and there has been interest from other hospitals within New Zealand and overseas.

We all can make a difference in the care of our patients, and we have a responsibility to do so. Be brave and bold, and step forward— no matter where you are on the nursing ladder.

• • •

Jenny Kendall is a nurse at Wellington Public Hospital, Capital and Coast District Health Board, Wellington, New Zealand.

Stacking the Cards in Our Favor

Ro Licata

Between 1998 and 2000 I was president of the nurses union—the Syndicat des Infirmieres et Infirmiers du Centre Universitaire de Sante McGill (SIICUSM)—at the Royal Victoria Hospital in Montreal, which is part of the of the McGill University Health Centre (MUHC). During this period, the union Executive and the Federation of Quebec nurses was active in addressing the problem of workplace violence. A 1995 survey conducted by the Federation of Quebec nurses (FIIQ) showed that 68 percent of respondents suffered physical assault, including being bitten, punched, or stabbed with a sharp object by patients, their family, or other staff. As part of the union's action plan, every international nurses' day, we would hold an event or activity, and our activities often focused on the issue of violence in the workplace. More and more nurses were breaking the silence about this issue.

One of the projects we held was to bring a women's group in to do self-defense teaching about how to respond to either a physical or psychological assault. In this group, we did a lot of role playing and held a lot of discussions. As we were sitting around in the discussion group with about fifty women present, someone mentioned the fact that when a nurse is assaulted, the reprimand is often directed at the nurse, the person who has been assaulted, not the person doing the assaulting. It's the classic "blaming the victim" tactic. The woman leading the session said that she'd always felt that the people who were assaulted should be giving something as a reprimand to the person doing the abuse.

This notion resonated with everyone, and we came up with the idea of giving out cards to people who were abusive in the hospital. We devised two cards: a pink one to keep and a red one that nurses could simply hand to anyone—patient, a patient's family member, a supervisor, a doctor, or even a coworker—in situations involving verbal abuse, disrespect, or threats. We printed up thousands of these pocket-sized cards and gave them out to nurses. The pink card said:

> I am empowering myself to eliminate violence in the workplace.
>
> 1. Take a deep breath; I trust myself.
> 2. Tell the person: "I do not accept this behavior" and give them the red card.
> 3. Report the incident to the hotline [a call-in number the union had established in collaboration with the employer].
> 4. Inform your union representative.

The red card was to be given to the abuser. It notified the person to whom it was handed that their "behavior is inappropriate as per the MUHC policy for the prevention of violence at work."

The first printing of three thousand cards was handed out within three months and the nurses were asking for more. We had cards in our union office, and nurses could pick them up there. We went around to the units to encourage union delegates on the units to distribute them and explain their use. We were always walking around the hospital talking to people about the cards. We also held information sessions around the cards. In these sessions we helped nurses learn what to say or do when they gave out a card. And we backed them up with follow-up investigations and complaints to management when they gave out a card or made a complaint.

Many nurses used the cards. Some told us that just knowing the cards existed helped them to be assertive and say something to the person without even giving them a card. Nurses often have a difficult time confronting threatening or abusive behavior. By giving them these cards, we gave them some way to deal with abuse that doesn't force them to confront it all by themselves. We were intent on making people understand that accepting this kind of behavior in the workplace was unacceptable. Just the act of handing out a card to someone was an assertion that nurses are important and they would no longer tolerate abuse in the workplace as part of their job description.

· · ·

Ro Licata, RN, has been a nurse for more than forty years. She has worked in critical care units in the United States and Canada and was president of SIICUSM from 1989–2008.

Part 2
WE DON'T HAVE TO EAT OUR YOUNG

Talk to any group of RNs, almost anywhere in the world, and you will eventually hear someone announce that "nurses eat their young." Aside from assertions that nursing is the "caring profession," this has become one of the profession's mantras. "We're our own worst enemies," they say. (This is in contrast to doctors, by the way, who they argue always support and stick up for one another).

To cite one example, I was just talking with a woman in her mid-fifties who had recently become a nurse. She'd left an important job—in which she'd had a lot of authority—to change careers. "In nursing school," she recounted, "I was really surprised to find that we were always told that nurses eat their young."

"Did you get any advice about how to deal with that?" I asked.

She shook her head. "No, they just told us it would happen, and that we shouldn't let it get to us. We should just," she paused and reflected, "I don't know what, ignore it, put up with it?"

I've come to believe that the constant repetition of this self-blaming mantra has had a pernicious effect on members of the profession. Repeat something often enough and you come to believe not only that it's true but also that it's inevitable. No wonder I find that so many RNs insist that nurses are somehow, by their very nature, incapable of nurturing and supporting each other. But I don't believe that for a minute. Sure, some RNs let each other down and even fail to welcome the new members of their profession who are still struggling to learn the ropes. But doctors can be bad team players too, even more adept at hazing, rather than mentoring, their "young." Just listen to a surgeon describe a dermatologist, or an internist lambaste those "damn specialists" who never return his or her phone calls.

If you believe that nurses are fated forever to turn against each other, read the stories in this section. Here you will meet nurses who went to bat for each other when they didn't have to; managers who came to the aid of hospital staff traumatized by an experience on the job; and nurse executives who put their own titles on the line to defend nursing budgets and services. In each story, mutual aid and protection—not cannibalism—prevailed.

Mentor Unto Others . . .

Clola Robinson-Blake

I've always hated starting a new job, especially the orientations, as a result of some not-so-pleasant experiences in the past. It didn't take me long to discover that my orientation for a new job on an oncology unit in a prominent hospital was going to be no different than the others. The orientation was all about business and the speed at which I was able to produce. But produce what? Better patient care? I wish.

The usual length of this orientation was six weeks and though that may sound like a long time, it flew by quickly. Throughout the entire six weeks, I was introduced to a field—oncology—that was new to me. Yet my fellow nurses didn't support me. Not at all. Instead, they bullied me, belittled me, and drove me far beyond my capabilities. Surviving this was only possible because I had many years of experience as a nurse and a strong determination to succeed. Fortunately for me, I completed my orientation before the six weeks was up and without a mishap.

I worked on this unit for many years and witnessed a rapid turnover rate among both RNs and nursing assistants. I think this happened for many reasons, but one was certainly the way my colleagues oriented nurses new to the unit.

When I finally became a preceptor (i.e., a senior staff who orients new staff to the unit functions and patient care), I was determined to do things differently. Although I followed the rules of orientation, I did not want new nurses to experience what I'd suffered and tried to help these recruits in a way that other nurses had not helped me.

My approach was—can you believe that this is unusual?—to treat my orientee with respect. I knew I had to fight any frustration I might experience and to understand that they were new graduates. My role

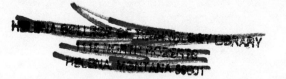

wasn't to sigh in exasperation because they didn't know something (how many times had I heard those sighs myself in my orientation). If they made a mistake, I didn't make them feel like dummies. After all, being new meant you would make mistakes, but you could learn from them. I was there to reassure them—to help them learn and to make them feel not only that we wanted but needed them to stay on the unit.

One day when I was orienting a new graduate, my colleagues and manager on the unit began to complain about the new orientee. They said she was too slow and didn't have enough knowledge. What was even worse, these nurses actually made derogatory comments in front of her.

During my encounters with this orientee, I found her to be very interested in her work. She was quite thorough (which takes time on a busy unit), willing to learn, and engaging. She was also empathetic to the patients and treated them with respect. I realized that with time she could become a valuable member of our team. Remembering the days when I was an orientee and wanted to quit because of the non-nurturing atmosphere on the unit, I decided to challenge these complaints.

I met with the manager of the unit and explained why I felt this orientee was a valuable addition to our unit. People who are new need time to grow and function more easily, I argued. I suggested that if veteran nurses treated her negatively, as they'd treated many others, they'd get negative results. The manager agreed with my argument and said we should give her a chance to prove herself. She also suggested that we meet with the other staff who assisted in her orientation. During this meeting, I was able to help my colleagues look at their styles of orientation and to take a more humane approach to a period in which people are vulnerable—especially new grads. There was no reason to set up a person to fail, we all concluded.

This nurse was successful in her orientation and became a valued member of the team on the oncology unit. She eventually became a preceptor herself and modeled a very different kind of behavior to the people she took under her wing than that which she and I had both experienced. Instead of eating our young on that unit, we began to actually nourish them.

. . .

CLOLA ROBINSON-BLAKE, RN, BSN, MS in Nursing (Clinical Specialist in Community Public Health), has worked in oncology nursing and has served as clinical faculty at the University of Maryland and Johns Hopkins School of Nursing.

A Dose of Diplomacy

Donna Schroeder

One busy day I was in charge of the medical intensive care unit. The unit is composed of sixteen beds, and acuity is often very high. Since we were down two nurses, the assignments were particularly challenging or even dangerous. Many of our patients were on ventilators and required a least one vocative infusion to support their blood pressure. Normally, such fragile patients would require their own nurse or at least be paired with another patient not as acutely ill. On this day, we were not able to accommodate this practice.

Over the course of the morning I overheard several nurses complaining that we seemed to have a lot of nurse managers on the unit and that they all seemed to be sitting at their desks at the back of the unit. They were right. Five nurses who serve within a management role were on the unit working on their usual paperwork.

It was often difficult to get nurse managers' help during busy times. Typically, charge nurses who requested this were told, "I'm sorry; I have to complete my own work today." Normally, I would walk around the unit seething rather than risk being turned down.

The behavior of management had always been puzzling to me and many other senior staff. Particularly since our health care system is known for the considerable number of errors that harm or kill patients every year. It would seem appropriate—indeed desirable—to discuss distribution of resources prior to the start of any shift to ensure safe practice. However, I can't think of any situation in recent memory when this has been done. Charge nurses are generally praised for "handling" the unit on such days. If a bedside nurse requests help, managers often tell her she isn't good at prioritizing. But how do you prioritize in this most impossible of situations?

Since I had recently taken a graduate-level course in teamwork, I decided to use one of the strategies discussed often in class. Instead of going up and berating or attacking the nurse managers, I would acknowledge their situation and then ask for help—not angrily demand it.

I approached one of the nurse managers and said, "Susan, I know how busy you are and how important your work is, but the staff could really use you're expertise at this time." I further explained to her that some of the assignments were particularly challenging, and the staff could use her leadership.

She left her paperwork and came on to the unit, spending several hours assisting staff with their assignments. At the end of the day, I approached her to say thank you. Then I explained the strategy I used in approaching her for assistance. By conveying appreciation for her expertise and acknowledging her role, the request had been delivered in a nonthreatening way. She thanked me and replied: "Donna, you don't know how many people come back here and yell, 'Get out here now and help us!' I really liked your approach."

Since that day I have practiced using this technique in many similar situations. Sometimes it works, but not always. What I have found most rewarding is that approaching the problem in this manner maintains a flow of communication between myself and the other party (not likely to happen if you are hostile and demanding), and it becomes easier to approach them and discuss these issues in more detail when there is more time. And guess what? It also feels a lot better this way. I guess it's what the Buddhists call mobilizing good karma.

· · ·

DONNA SCHROEDER, RN, MSN, works as a critical care nurse; her degree is in Nursing and Health Policy and she is currently enrolled in the University of Maryland at Baltimore program for Critical Care and Trauma Nurse Practitioner.

Standing Up for What You Don't Know

Judy Schaefer

I could have lost my job. I remember vividly, still, after more than thirty years. A scared new graduate nurse in a university teaching hospital, and I stood up for my patients, my profession, and myself. I was thrilled to have this job and would never have suspected that this risky situation would arise, especially around the joy and happy background music of the holidays.

I was a graduate nurse in my first job, and it was my first holiday on the medical-surgical ward. I was learning and struggling to keep up, as was one of my classmates. Nurses were asked to request days off months before Christmas and New Years, decorations were being hung by night shift nurses, and music was starting to fill the air during the day and evening. As the holiday neared, there was discussion about getting patients discharged, closing one of the wings, and giving nurses time off so they could be with their families. Senior nurses, according to the policy, would get first choice of days off.

On the day before the Christmas and New Year holiday schedule went into effect, I came onto the ward, took report, and walked toward the med room to prepare my meds. The clinical manager came to me and told me that I would be "charge" nurse tomorrow and the next couple days. "Okay?" she asked. She had complete faith in me, she said, and had been pleased with my performance these first months. My classmate, a novice like myself, would also be on my team. Because the senior nurses, per policy, had first choice, there would be no senior nurses on the floor over the holidays.

Before I answered her, I had a vision: All the beds down all those wings were filled with my mother, clones and clones of my dear mother. All those beds contained patients who were seriously ill in this university trauma center hospital, which was swarming with medical students, interns, residents, and attendings who seemed to delight in writing conflicting orders—at least that's the way it seemed to me as a new graduate. My risky but assertive decision came from a place that I did not know or recognize. Without thinking, I blurted out, "I cannot come on the unit tomorrow and take on the duty of charge nurse."

"Where did that come from? Who said that?" I wondered. I had just refused duty! My two feet were flat to the floor and my back straight as the proverbial stick. My hands were shaking, so I clasped them behind my back. Perspiration was already pooling in the small of my back. My unscented deodorant was failing my underarms. I had just put my new job at risk. I loved this job. I needed this job. What the hell was I doing? Didn't I want to rise to the occasion? Be smart? Look smart?

The clinical manager insisted that I was capable of doing the job. I countered that I was a graduate nurse and not ready.

She continued to insist that I could do the job.

I reminded her that my teammate was a graduate nurse and also not prepared to undertake these duties.

While I was sure I was doing the right thing, it terrified me to do it. Refusing duty? Insubordination? What kind of nurse was I? Couldn't I apply the scientific principles that I had been taught and react appropriately to handle emergencies as they arose?

In retrospect, had I accepted the assignment, everything would *probably* have been all right. *Maybe* I could have muddled along successfully for a few days. But what if we had an emergency that, as a novice nurse, I couldn't have handled? Is dumb luck a good enough standard of care? I didn't have to find out. Not then.

Although I expected some backlash, my clinical manager's thoughts appeared to start spinning right in front of me. She became quiet and thoughtful. I was not reprimanded. There was no retaliation from my colleagues. I perceived then and now that I was taken seriously. In fact, I suspect that my stand reminded them that there was a different way to look at the holiday scheduling policy; that certain institutional liabilities must be considered. I kept my job and thrived that year. The holiday situation was reversed, and a more senior nurse was scheduled to work with us as charge nurse for the week.

In discussing this situation years later over a glass of wine with a nursing colleague, she jokingly agreed that, yes, this kind of clarity in leadership skill and clinical skill is important: "If you aren't careful, all of a sudden you are the leader of a bunch of idiots going blindly down the wrong happy road together."

As I consider my thirty-plus-year career, I realize that I have remained a safe practitioner by being very clear about what I know and don't know. Which in both cases is a lot.

• • •

JUDY SCHAEFER, RNC, MA, is the editor of *The Poetry of Nursing: Poems and Commentaries of Leading Nurse-Poets* and coeditor of *Between the Heartbeats.*

Broken Bones and Ice Cream

Edie Brous

Emergency department (ED) nurses become toughened after time. The relentless exposure to human tragedy would take its toll if we did not develop defenses. We learn to cope with an endless parade of suffering humanity. We develop thicker skins through use of gallows humor and even pride ourselves on our emotional calluses. We believe nothing surprises us. We can handle anything thrown at us. We believe we have seen it all. You cannot startle or shock us (or so we think). We are ED nurses. We are strong. Hear us roar.

With calm professionalism, we tend to patients with gunshot wounds, horrific motor vehicle accident injuries, sudden strokes and heart attacks, gastrointestinal hemorrhages, and seizures. We matter-of-factly change clothes when we are splashed with blood, bile, vomit, or urine. We see gruesome things that would make the average person faint. Violence, trauma, devastating diseases, and death are part of our daily work lives. We support the rape survivor but do not go home in tears. We feel compassion for the crime victim but do not leave the job in fear. We are exposed to gore and horror but it does not give us nightmares. We ED nurses are a tough bunch. It should be impossible to get to us. But it is not. At times we must fight against our own self-image to take care of ourselves. We each have that one experience that will pierce those calluses and shake us to the core. For me and my ED colleagues, this experience took the form of a battered child.

I was the nursing manager of a busy New York City ED one March morning when a child I will call "Allen" broke our hearts. At six years of age, he was rushed into our ED with catastrophic injuries. Despite frantic efforts throughout the entire morning, we were forced to pronounce him dead around noon. My staff was devastated.

We knew Allen. We had treated this little boy on multiple occasions and always reported our concerns to authorities. Repeatedly, this battered child presented with escalating injuries, and each time we attempted to prevent his return to such a dangerous home. But again and again, the court returned him to his abusive parents in the name of "keeping families together." We had done everything possible to prevent this, but now he was dead.

When the alarm bells went off when we first developed an index of suspicion, and at every subsequent visit, we identified our concerns to social services. Social services consistently reported to protective services. Protective services always appealed to the court. Yet the system kept returning this child to people who physically battered and terrorized him. Every nurse in the ED knew that he had to be removed from this home before it was too late. We knew he would come to us "permanently horizontal" one day if he was not protected. And now that day had arrived.

After pronouncing death, we sent his little body to radiology for a mandated long-bone survey (a full, head-to-toe x-ray study). We shuddered when we discovered the sheer number of fractures in different stages of healing. Clearly this boy had known nothing in his short life except pain and fear.

The primary nurse (I'll call her "Mary") assigned to him had a daughter of the same age and was clearly shaken. She was scheduled to work until 3:00 p.m. I had called an evening shift nurse and requested that she come in a little early, which she agreed to do. When she arrived, I asked her to relieve Mary and have her come to see me. At 1:00, Mary approached me and asked where I wanted her to go now that she had endorsed her district to the evening nurse. She was an ED nurse, ready to keep on working. But I knew that, in this case, I had to fight her own self-image in order to protect her.

"Home," I responded, "Go home and hug your child."

Mary looked surprised and said she was scheduled to work until three.

"Not today—I will pay you for the full shift, but I want you to go hug your child because that is what all of us need you to do."

"But my daughter is in school," she protested.

"So take her out. Tell the school you have a personal situation and you are picking her up for the day. Then hug her to pieces and play jacks, color in coloring books together—something, anything. When you come in tomorrow I want you to tell us how you spent the afternoon. It will be healing for us. *We* need you to do this."

Mary left for the day and we continued saving lives and stamping out disease, as we like to say. But a heavy cloud covered the ED as we went about our duties. The enthusiasm was gone. The light-hearted jokes, joviality, and protective cynicism were gone. We were vulnerable. Our defenses had failed us. I wondered how long this would last.

Psychiatric nurse specialists conducted "debriefing" sessions that were attended by nurses, physicians, unit secretaries, registration clerks, paramedics, even housekeeping. The entire team had been traumatized and needed camaraderie for comfort. We met the next day and discussed our futile efforts to save Allen's life, the emotions that engendered, and our difficulty in dealing with them. Though hardened by years or even decades of ED experiences, most of us openly wept. Some sobbed uncontrollably.

Then Mary joined the session. Everyone fell silent as she took her seat.

"Yesterday," she started, "I called my daughter's school and told them I would be picking her up early. When I got to the school, she was surprised to see me and asked what was wrong. I thought I had been hiding my distress, but she picked up on it. I decided to share it with her. I told her Mommy had a bad day at work and was very sad. I told her I needed some special, stolen time with her and I wanted to do something fun with her to cheer up. Leave it to a six year old to have the answer. She gave me a huge 'cheer up hug' followed by her prescription. 'You need ice cream, Mommy! That always makes us feel better.'"

"So ice cream it was. We went to the Dairy Queen, got cones, and took them to the park. We sat on a park bench together, and I listened to her chatter about everything and nothing for the rest of the afternoon. I kept looking at her and saying to myself, 'She is safe. She is loved. She is happy. She is alive.' We held hands on the walk home, and I knew that this would be one treasured moment from her childhood that I would remember always. I hope she will as well."

We hope so, too, Mary, because hearing how you spent your afternoon helped us to carry on. And carry on we did. After all, we are ED nurses.

. . .

EDIE BROUS, RN Esq., is a nurse attorney specializing in medical malpractice defense litigation, professional licensure, representation, and nursing advocacy.

Treating Transition Shock

Judy Boychuk Duchscher

"Judy, just get your degree—you can 'make a difference' later" was the unexpected mantra that echoed from a surprising number of my nursing colleagues as I embarked on what would be a six-year commitment to my doctoral studies in nursing. In 1996, I had entered my Master of Nursing program, curious about findings that suggested new nurses leave their basic nursing program with the ability to apply an analytical approach to their practice as nurses but within months of being introduced into the "real" world, they become prescriptive "doers." As I engaged in my own graduate research, I discovered that the motivations for this change could in part be attributed to subtle messages from their disenfranchised colleagues (nurses and physicians) that in order to "fit in" these new practitioners had to accept the embedded traditions of their workplaces, complete their required tasks on time without questioning the rationale behind them, and refrain from challenging the status quo. They learned to "follow orders" and assume the "busy" work that they perceived as preventing them from actually "nursing." Subsequently, these idealistic and motivated graduates developed a sense of disconnect between what they were being told about their duties as a nurse and what they had been educated to understand was the role of a professional nurse. I wanted to understand more about what might be motivating this "back-peddling," what might be happening to the theory, professional standards, and practice ethics these neophytes had been taught, and how they were making sense of these apparent contradictions. To accomplish this, I followed up my graduate work with doctoral studies in the area of professional role transition for new nurses.

By 2007, I had finished my doctorate in nursing and built a strong base of research and study on how nurses make their initial transition into the professional world after being students. I was able to generate two theoretical models, the first of which outlined the stages of transition through which new nursing graduates progress during their initial year in practice. I hoped this model would provide a framework for educators and employers to understand and implement supportive strategies for these young nurses that could move them along a productive career path with a minimal amount of professional tension. I have come to believe that it is not possible, nor desirable, to expect that the process of moving from school to professional work will be uneventful; this period encompasses tremendous growth for a new professional and with that growth necessarily comes pain. Our task, as their supporters, is to determine what we can and cannot do to reduce the difficulty in this process and then put strategies in place that either take away the obstacles to successful professional integration or provide support to get through the rough spots that everyone experiences when going through a major change in their lives.

The second model that arose from my work I labeled "transition shock," as this was the most accurate term I was able to think of to describe the initial few months of transition for new nurses moving from school to work. Rather than feeling welcomed by the experienced nurses they "look up to" or being embraced for the contemporary knowledge they bring to practice, these new recruits describe a professional culture that resists their ideas and places obstacles in their way as they try to enact change in their workplaces. Over time, these energetic new nurses feel disappointed and then disillusioned by their lack of involvement in decision making about patient care, the level of apathy and even hostility in the experienced colleagues who are supposed to be their role models and mentors, and the general dysfunction of the health care system that consistently underuses and misappropriates their capability and disempowers them as they try to advocate for patient needs and apply their professional knowledge and skill.

So I had my theory in hand. But I knew that wasn't enough. I wanted my work to amount to more than an exhaustive literature collection or carefully constructed theoretical models gathering dust on a shelf. And so, during the end years of my doctoral work I brought together a team of new nurses and launched the concept of a national network to support new nurses during the first year of their transition from being students to being professional practitioners. I admit that the germination of this plan emerged equally out of my own personal experiences as a patient and then as a family member within the hospital system.

As I met for the first time with this dynamic young group of graduates who had been prior students of mine, my father lay dying in a neighboring city. Ironically, it was his birthday. My father's subsequently premature death was a defining period in my life—I often think of it now as his final gift to me. As I stood over his bedside several days before he died, I swore I would never enter another hospital. A profound sense of emptiness originated out of a powerlessness that overwhelmed me as I reflected on the medical mishaps that ultimately resulted in his death. Even after thirty years of navigating the hospital hierarchy as a nurse, I was unable to prevent my father from living out his final days caught in the cracks of the broken institution we call health "care." My father died of multisystem failure by every definition! I watched helplessly as communication among disciplines fractured, leaving my father a victim of missed diagnoses and "too little too late" interventions. I watched experienced nurses so busy "following orders" that they were unable to detect the signs of his acute myocardial infarction as it evolved before their eyes. I saw new graduates moving patients from room to room to accommodate the changing census, and managers spending valuable time working as "staffing clerks" while *everyone* failed to notice that my father's potassium was 5.5 and that they were still delivering K+ through his IV. I saw battles for power replace concerns for patient welfare, and I witnessed the ultimate outcome of a failure to fully engage the knowledge, insight, and skill of the nursing role. But this time it was personal.

After witnessing yet another failure of a system eroding under the weight of chronic organizational and human resource mismanagement, I was even more determined to support the newest members of our profession to *be* the change that the nursing profession had always represented for me. The answer was starting a new organization, Nursing the Future, which served as the vehicle for that support. To start the organization, I joined with a group of like-minded and motivated newly graduated nurses and acquired a small grant from our provincial Ministry of Health in Saskatchewan, allowing us to move ahead with a plan to provide a network of resources to new graduates and those who supported them. This network grew quickly as the resources we created resonated with the immediate needs of these novice practitioners. Using my research as a framework, we designed a one hundred page manual that outlined the stages of transition and provided tips for dealing with the issues related to establishing one's self as a professional nurse—for example, on coping with stress, adjusting to shift-work, dealing with a dying patient, working with physicians and senior nursing staff, and managing a complex nursing workload.

My team and I spoke at nursing schools and conferences across Canada. We introduced graduates to the experienced nurses and more seasoned graduates who would mentor and encourage them. As the organization evolved, we initiated a website (www.nursingthe future.ca), hosted support groups for regional graduates to interact with each other, and developed an e-newsletter that featured graduates and seasoned nurses who were making a difference in their workplaces. In this way, we provided new nurses with the resources and support they would need to stand up for their professional practice standards and ethics and move forward with their creative ideas for practice improvements even when faced with opposition.

The process of starting and growing this organization met with considerable resistance from some well-meaning but out-of-touch colleagues who told me to "worry about that later." I heard from senior practice nurses who struggled to understand why young nurses would need this support when clearly this had never been available "when we were starting out"—as though the absence of a needed resource for us should dictate withholding it from them. Over the years, I have come to believe that the greatest challenge for nursing is the profession itself. It seems we have arrived at a place where our energies are more focused on the way things have become—the protocols and routines—rather than on examining our traditions and making the changes necessary for nurses to practice to the level of our education and capability. We allow ourselves to be pitted against one other in the camps of practice and theory as though one is possible without the other. We divide ourselves around the issue of scope of practice as if we all didn't need each other. Despite the ongoing concerns about the inadequate supply of nursing human resources to manage the existing workloads in direct care, nurses themselves resist relinquishing particular tasks that do not require their level of intellect or practice skill. At the same time, nurses are being asked to hand over to nonlicensed staff duties that require more experience and theoretical knowledge than is recognized; what direct-care nurses "do" is so highly integrated that the skill we use is almost invisible, for example, knowing that a patient is getting a severe hospital-acquired infection such as *C. difficile* based on the smell emanating from the bathroom.

As we continue to develop our group, we are heartened by the stories of the new graduates whose early professional experiences are made easier by our support. Now, when I hear my seasoned colleagues lament that "we never had support like this," I gain a greater appreciation for Dr. Phil's adage "And how's that been workin' for ya"? To anyone who believes passionately that the quality of health care depends on the ability of our young nurses to be valued for what they offer, I say do something, *anything* . . . just don't do nothing. For me, starting at the beginning made the most sense.

• • •

Judy Boychuk Duchscher, RN, BScN, MN, PhD, is the Founder and Executive Director of Nursing the Future and Assistant Professor, Faculty of Nursing, University of Calgary, Alberta, Canada.

The Empty-Hands Round

Amaia Sáenz de Ormijana

I was called in for a four-month job as a staff nurse at a medical ward in an acute care hospital in the Basque Country, Spain, where I live. The ward for thirty-two patients was divided into sixteen double rooms. There were two nurses and two assistants on the unit on every shift. Both nurses and assistants followed the same shift-rotation, so they usually worked with the same people on each shift.

Each nurse, along with the assistant, was in charge of sixteen patients, one of them holding responsibility for the care of patients in rooms 1 through 8 and the other one for patients in rooms 9 through 16. It was a very busy ward, with an average patient age of eighty-two, and lots of calls for pain medication.

My colleague, Sandra (names and identifying details have been changed to protect confidentiality), had been working in this unit for six years. She was fourteen years older than me. She was a registered nurse and had been trained at a school of nursing where technical knowledge and skills were highly valued.

Our institution tried to offer a holistic approach to nursing care, where health was understood as much more than the absence of illness. In reality, caring for sixteen acute patients during an eight-hour shift did not leave us with too many opportunities to go beyond patients' physical care. On our shifts together, Sandra was in charge of patients in rooms 1 through 8, and I was in charge of the other half.

In addition to my initial nursing three-year diploma training in Spain, I had had the opportunity to travel, study (BScN, MSc), and work abroad, and so I was used to doing what I now call the "empty-hands round"; that is, walking into patients' rooms with nothing in my hands, with the single goal being to introduce myself to patients ("I'm Amaia Sáenz de Ormijana, the nurse in charge of your care today"). I do this at the beginning of every shift and explain to them that I will be available to them for the rest of the shift ("I will be here until ten o'clock and, although I will be coming by every now and then, please do not hesitate to call me in case you need anything that you think I can help you with"). I follow this with an emphasis on pain control strategies ("Please, let me know about your pain as soon as you start feeling it; the sooner you take the medication, the easier it will be to get the pain under control and the quicker you will feel better"). Frequently, patients would already know me from previous shifts. In this case, I would just walk in, call them by their names, and ask them about their day so far and their worries or concerns regarding their health and well-being. I would do this as soon as I had listened to previous-shift colleagues' report on patients and before starting the "real" work of preparing medication, measuring blood pressures, getting patients out of bed, or admitting patients from the emergency room, to name a few of the activities carried out on a regular shift. I would thus walk in the rooms with my hands empty.

This empty-hands round of mine was not at all common among nurses in this hospital, nor in many other institutions in Spain. As I was a "novice nurse," having worked for three years then, I remember feeling embarrassed for doing this routine due to unpleasant comments from colleagues. Most of them waited for a call from a patient in need before initiating contact with that patient. After a few days in the unit though, my attitude changed, and I somehow found the strength to do things the way I thought I had to, according to my professional values and my understanding of what is good for patients.

And so, after a few days working with Sandra in the unit and feeling she was respectful with my way of seeing and understanding "the health care world," I decided to start doing my "empty-hands round" again in this new setting.

About two weeks later, Sandra made a comment regarding the workload distribution in our shift: "You really are a lucky girl, Amaia. I have been thinking that lately the patients you are responsible for seem to be a lot 'lighter' than mine because they do not ring the bell as often as mine do."

I did not agree with her explanation of the "phenomenon" but was not brave enough to tell her about my hypothesis that my empty-hands round rather than patient acuity was the variable factor. Instead,

I told her I'd be glad to switch the rooms assigned to us. She would be in charge of the patients in the last eight rooms, and I would be responsible for those in rooms 1 through 8. The first time I offered, she rejected my suggestion, but a week later she accepted it: "There is not much to lose by trying it," she said.

After another couple of weeks during which I was in charge of the so-called "heavier" patients, bingo, the same thing happened again. I would do my empty-hands round every time I would start my shift, and it seemed that "my" patients would ring the bell much less often than those Sandra was caring for. We never counted the number of calls, but Sandra agreed that, again, I was getting fewer calls from patients under my care than she was.

One late shift, as we were having our break, she said, "Amaia, this change we made in the rooms assigned to each of us has not worked. Once again I seem to be getting the heavier patient load and that just does not make any sense. I have been thinking about it for a couple of days and I think I have the answer: It is not a matter of how sick they are or what a care-load they have. Your patients' ringing the bell less often than mine has to do with the fact that they feel more secure and more closely watched when you introduce yourself to them and assure them you will be here for their care all shift long."

She asked me for help. She wanted to do something about the way she "nursed" her patients but, at the same time, admitted she was not capable of introducing herself to patients. She had been trained in a different way of nursing and so introducing herself to patients was not within her scope of practices. She wanted to incorporate that into her practice but lacked the personal tools, abilities, or strategies to start doing so. She did decide, however, that she would try walking into her patients' rooms with empty hands to talk to them. The next day she began this new practice.

Some months after, I met Sandra for coffee. I was no longer working on the unit, and Sandra was now, as she put it, working with a nurse very similar to the old-her. She had had to listen to some disparaging comments about her empty-hands round. People asked her if she thought she would be better paid for doing this and insisted it was just a waste of time. Finally she had stopped doing it. She did not feel comfortable going back to her old behavior, she said, but felt she could not buck the peer pressure she experienced: "It is a matter of personal survival, Amaia," she confessed.

In my opinion, Sandra was very smart, honest, and brave to share her thoughts with me. But alone, with no shared culture to support her, the status quo prevailed. But not for me. I know this helps my patients and is part of my professional practice. My empty-hands rounds will continue.

• • •

AMAIA SÁENZ DE ORMIJANA, RN, BScHs, MSc, has worked for over five years at different hospital units in the Basque Public Health Service, Spain.

Part 3

EXCUSE ME, DOCTOR, YOU'RE WRONG

We've heard the unfortunate stories of how nurses can abuse or mistreat other nurses. Some argue they do this because they've been so badly treated by doctors. Horizontal violence is the logical consequence of vertical violence, the argument goes. Whatever the reason for the parlous state of nurse–nurse relationships, it's clear that the state of nurse–doctor relationships needs a lot of improvement. When I first went into hospitals to observe nurses, I was impressed—*depressed* is perhaps a better word—by the way doctors treated nurses as well as by the way so many nurses adapted to— rather than protested—that treatment. It seemed like the women's movement had bypassed nursing (or nursing had bypassed the women's movement) and that this predominantly female profession seemed to accept behavior that wouldn't be tolerated in other professional workplaces.

The toxic hierarchies that one sees in the health care system are the result of tensions and conflicts that have existed between medicine and nursing ever since the mid-nineteenth century, when nursing emerged as the first mass profession for respectable women. Doctors were, at the same time, moving into hospitals in large numbers, where they soon gained control over nursing practice. To this day, some doctors continue to view nurses only as the handmaidens of medicine or, in the current jargon, "physician extenders" or "allied health professionals." Because nurses lack an MD degree, too many physicians fail to recognize nurses' valuable knowledge and skills.

Of course, there are many physicians and nurses who work well together. In the course of their work, however, nurses repeatedly encounter doctors who were, as one doctor explains, "taught how to give orders to nurses, not to talk to them." The stories in this section show how nurses get around the socialization of both medicine and nursing. These RNs, like many others, have found interesting and innovative ways to get doctors to rethink and reject such shortsighted attitudes. When physicians persist in their bad behavior, these nurses do not back off. In the process, they make patients safer by reducing dysfunction at the intersection of nursing and medicine and help lay the foundation for the kind of teamwork that is essential if we are to keep patients safe and make the health care workplace a far less toxic and frustrating environment for all.

Eye/I Advocacy

Jane Black

Nurses who work in the emergency department interact with the ED's own doctors day in and day out. You come to know and trust these doctors, become familiar with their habits, and learn how best to approach each when issues come up with written orders. Working with ED doctors is also great because you don't have to call them up—they are right there! If you need an order or want to discuss a patient's care with them, it is an easy task; no calling the paging service, no waiting for a reply, no putting up with annoyed doctors whom you've interrupted with your question or request.

Sometimes, however, private physicians come to see their patients in the ED, and working with private physicians in the ED can be more challenging. One afternoon I was taking care of an eighty-four-year-old man being seen by his private cardiologist. The patient had presented with intermittent chest pain. After a few tests to assure himself that the patient was not in any acute danger, the physician wrote some orders and left the hospital. Did he check with me, the nurse? Discuss his plan? Solicit my input? No.

At the bedside, I began to discuss with the gentleman the drug I was left orders to administer to him: enoxaparin sodium. The drug is an anticoagulant. It reduces the ability of the blood to clot, thereby decreasing the risk of a heart attack, which typically is caused by a clot blocking the flow of blood to the heart muscle.

"I take ICaps," the patient told me.

"Oh?" I said, "What are you taking those for?" I knew that ICaps were a vitamin formula sold for eye health.

"I have some problems with my vision," he said. With further probing, I learned not just that he had decreased eyesight but also that the patient had a history of retinal hemorrhage. The blood vessels at the back of his eyes were fragile and prone to leak or bleed, causing loss of vision. Administering an anticoagulant to this patient could potentially result in catastrophic retinal bleeding.

I held the drug and put out a call to the physician. "I'm calling about the order for enoxaparin. The patient has a history of retinal hemorrhage," I told him. The shudder on the other end of the phone was nearly palpable, and the doctor stammered out, "Don't give it to him!" Well, I'd already decided that. The fear in the physician's voice turned into relief as I explained that I had not given the drug, but he never did thank me for catching his dangerous error.

I don't suppose this incident stands out for its excitement or drama, but I believe that I saved this patient's eyesight. It reminds me not to become complacent about physician's orders, to take the time to think orders through, talk to and listen to the patient, and not to assume the physician has thought of everything.

· · ·

JANE BLACK, RN, MS, has been a practicing nurse since graduating from the University of Arizona in 1983. Her clinical background includes critical care, trauma, and emergency nursing.

As If the Patient Can Hear You

Clarke Doty

Because nurses refer to themselves as "patient advocates," it may seem like we're born knowing how to advocate. That's hardly the case. In fact, I can remember the first time I felt a strong sense of duty to defend *my* patient, the first time I felt—and acted—like a patient advocate.

I was a nursing student in one of my earliest medical-surgical clinical practicums. I was working in a small hospital, caring for an elderly patient who'd had a stroke. She couldn't speak and one side of her body was paralyzed, but her eyes were open and she seemed alert when I walked into her room for the first time. I introduced myself, explained I was a nursing student, and talked to her while I examined her. I listened with my stethoscope and told her what I heard. I told her about each part of my assessment. She made eye contact at times. I wondered if she could understand me. I imagined how terrifying it would feel to be unable to communicate with the outside world, utterly trapped, and I couldn't help but hope that, if recovery wasn't possible for her, she might at least be spared the awfulness of a conscious mind locked inside a failing body.

As I continued assessing the patient and charting, a man who looked to be in his early seventies and dressed in a brown suit entered the room. I looked up from the chart and watched as he took the stethoscope from around his neck and performed a quick assessment of the patient. Not once did he speak to her. He finally looked over at me, gestured for me to hand him the chart, and said, "I'm going to order some Lasix for the edema." He then walked out of the room, taking the chart with him.

I followed him into the hall where he stood writing in the patient's chart. I introduced myself. "You're not the nurse?" he asked, without looking up. "No, but I'll let her know about the Lasix," I replied. He placed the chart in the box next to the patient's door (rather than return it to me). Then, speaking without thinking, before he could walk off, I said, "How do you know she can't hear or understand you?" This time he looked at me. "She isn't brain dead, but she is unable to respond or follow commands," he stated simply.

"But perhaps it might be more respectful to address the patient herself rather than talk about her like she's not even in the room," I blurted. ("*And* knock before you enter a patient's room, *and* introduce yourself, *and* try asking politely for a chart as opposed to impatient hand gestures," I added silently.) His brow furrowed for a moment before he turned and walked back down the hall without saying a word.

Fuming, I went back into my patient's room. I explained about the Lasix. I looked for signs of comprehension. She gazed at the bed railing. Later that day, when my clinical instructor called me over, my heart pounded as I realized I might be reprimanded for my impudence, but she only wanted to hand back some graded paperwork. I never got any feedback from the doctor.

Thinking back on that time, I can laugh a little at my indignant outburst, the totally inexperienced nursing student scolding the seventy-year-old attending physician. But I'm so glad I said something. It was not only the right thing but the only thing to do.

• • •

CLARKE DOTY, RN, BSN, has worked in thoracic oncology at Memorial Sloan Kettering Cancer Center and in women's services at Duke University Medical Center. She is currently working in the Emergency Department at Duke and is pursuing an MSN in Nursing Education at Duke University's School of Nursing.

Don't Just Add Nurses and Stir

Janet Rankin

In the fall of 2008, the Canadian federal government mandated that all schools of nursing and medicine across Canada establish curricula activities to bring nursing and medical students together during their education. The government did this because of concerns about teamwork—or the lack of it—and safe patient care.

As representative of the faculty of nursing in my university, I volunteered to talk with the faculty of medicine to plan strategies to deal with this new mandate. I met with the person from the faculty of medicine who was responsible for moving this initiative forward. We sat down and began to brainstorm about finding time to bring the students together across the two very crowded programs.

"What do you know about the medical school program?" the woman asked me.

"Very little," I said.

She proceeded to describe the amount of course work the medical faculty crammed into only three years. The take-home message was that it would be really tough to merge our classes. Our first-year nursing students enter in September, while their program starts four weeks earlier. Right from the start just coordinating scheduling seemed like an insurmountable barrier.

As if this wasn't bad enough, as our meeting progressed, she told me that she had been consulting with the teaching faculty and acknowledged that there was some resistance to developing a collaboration with the nursing program. Nonetheless, she said she had identified three "early adopters," teachers who would be open to having student nurses join their medical school classes.

This agreement, however, seemed based on an assumption that nursing students would join activities that already existed in the medical curriculum. For example, student nurses, she said, could join medical students during a second-year simulation exercise around a pediatric case that the medical school had already developed. "Couldn't we develop a case together?" I queried. That didn't seem possible.

Another idea was for student nurses to join the medical students in a large lecture class given by the health authority about patient safety issues. I questioned the utility of nursing and medical students attending a joint lecture. I wondered how people could develop a foundation for interprofessional relationships and communication simply by sitting next to each other. She laughingly agreed, saying, "Yes, we don't want to make this a dating service," an odd comment given that 50 percent of medical school classes are made up of women.

She seemed to believe that the best way to proceed was to connect the students once they were well established within their respective disciplinary courses of study. I suggested that the students meet one another early in their professional education before they were initiated into the roles and expectations of the health care hierarchy.

How about convening a class where all the students could mingle in small groups to talk about their expectations of nursing and medical work? I suggested. This way we could identify and address some of the myths that become entrenched as students progress through their respective programs. I was also clear that any simulated activities that the students engaged in should be developed to address real issues that arise among nurses and doctors in the workplace. We should work together to create scenarios specifically for this purpose. For example, I wondered whether a simulation regarding doctors' orders might be useful. The woman told me that there is no formal class or discussion about doctors' orders in their highly "integrated" curriculum.

The message I got during this first meeting was that if student nurses and medical students were to get together, the medical program could only accommodate us within *their* established schedule. There was no time in the medical curriculum design to address the important task of learning about one another's work and developing insight into how physicians and nurses might collaborate more effectively. The attitude seemed to be "add nurses and stir" (or don't even stir)! This was not to be a joint culinary project in which we developed the recipes, tested them together, and then invited our students to partake. Medicine was graciously giving us the prepackaged condensed soup and suggesting we could add a little seasoning to their culinary creation. It was clear that, in future meetings, I would have to confront many challenges. How could I convince the medical school community that spending some time and effort to design a way that nursing and medical students might better understand one another's work as it relates to patient care is actually worth it?

Nurses care about this issue because it's such a problem for us and we recognize it's a problem for our patients. Even though so many doctors I know do care immensely about nurse–physician communication and its impact on patients, it's most often expressed as a private, not an official, concern. Now it had become official. But even though we knew about the importance of teamwork to patient safety and there were now resources available to support this initiative, it was not easy to narrow the great divide between medicine and nursing.

As I left that meeting I recognized that in our subsequent discussions, I would need to "sell" medicine on the benefits of working with nurses. Medical students have many important things to learn, as do nursing students, but when the rubber hits the road and they have to deal with one another, all their knowledge and technical proficiency may be overwhelmed by the fact that they have no idea how to function on a real team—and patients die as a result.

I am happy to report that in the successive meetings with the faculty of medicine, I added a little heat to the soup. I insisted that medicine and nursing are *both* key ingredients. If we combined our joint strengths and gave a good stir, we could nourish both ourselves and our patients. We are now developing activities to teach nursing students and medical students how to work as effective teams. It seems as though we are actually cooking collaboratively.

· · ·

Janet Rankin, RN, PhD, is the coauthor of *Managing to Nurse: Inside Canada's Health Care Reform*, Assistant Professor at the University of Calgary School of Nursing, and is an institutional ethnographer.

Gloves Off

Nancy Marie Valentine

As a new chief nurse leader in a busy city hospital, I took time to break into the inner-city culture. The cadre of nurses I was working with could, on one hand, be as kind as any I had ever encountered. As I witnessed their care, they could literally bring tears to my eyes. On the other hand, they could be tough as nails because they had seen it all.

One day, I knew I had started to gain their trust when the "take no prisoners" head nurse of the surgical intensive care unit, Mary, called my office for an emergency appointment. Mary came storming into my office as furious as I had ever seen her. With eyes blazing, she started to sputter out her anger with the medical director of surgical services, Dr. H., who had a reputation for being very difficult to deal with in a variety of settings. Mary reported that the day before, he had approached a patient on her unit and, with his *bare hands*, examined an open surgical wound, removing dead tissue with his fingers! When she confronted him, he told her it was his patient and she should not interfere with his judgment.

Calming her down, I agreed that his behavior—touching an open wound with bare hands—was unacceptable and suggested that we meet with him together. I also suggested that the patient be seen by the infection control team. She agreed to both, and the meeting with Dr. H occurred a few days later. Dr. H. was asked why he had not taken the usual precautions and used gloves? He declared that this was a better way of getting to feel the wound. He further defended his actions by insisting that this technique was described in the literature.

That's most interesting, I told him. I'd love to see a copy of the article. Could he produce that for us? I asked. He said he would and left the meeting in a rush. Of course we never saw any such article.

We reported the incident to the medical director, and Dr. H. was instructed to use gloves on all patients thereafter. This incident and aftermath, of course, did not cure Dr. H. of his impetuous behavior. It did, however, put him on notice that the nursing organization was prepared to take action if and when his behavior was potentially harmful to patients.

• • •

NANCY MARIE VALENTINE, RN, PhD, DSc (HON), MSN, MPH, FAAN, FNAP, is a psychiatric nurse by clinical training, former Director of Nursing at Boston City Hospital, Vice President for Nursing at McLean Hospital, Belmont, Mass., and national CNO, U.S. Department of Veterans Affairs, Washington, D.C., and is currently Senior Vice President and CNO at Main Line Health, Bryn Mawr, Pennsylvania.

The Overlooked Symptom

Jo Stecher

I came to work that morning and had two patients in our transplant intensive care unit. One was a twenty-two-year-old man who had received a liver transplant about forty-eight hours earlier. When I was doing my morning head-to-toe check, I found that he was very sleepy, his eyes were closed, he was jaundiced, and he wouldn't respond when I talked to him. When he did try to talk to me, he mumbled incomprehensibly.

I knew these symptoms were a problem. As an experienced transplant nurse, I knew that when you give somebody a liver and it works, they're not jaundiced and they're alert. They're perky, eating, talking, and even walking the halls.

This young man was doing none of that. So I checked all his vital signs, his blood pressure, pulse, temperature. Everything was where it should have been at that point in time, two days post transplant. Although his urine output was okay, the urine was a dark amber color—which was a concern. I did his morning lab work, and everything was fine. But I was still worried. As the shift progressed, he became more lethargic and sleepy. I did another set of blood work on him, and it started to document that life in his liver was deteriorating. His urine output was now a very thick sludge that was brown colored and basically unmeasureable as a liquid.

I paged the resident, who blew me off with some comment like, "I'm the doctor," and so I shouldn't worry. I told him bluntly that I was worried and that I was going to talk to the chief resident, and he said, "No don't call the chief resident. I think it's all right, but I'm going to keep an eye on him." To which I replied, "I am, too."

A few hours later, when I became more concerned because the patient was even more unresponsive, I paged the resident again and got the same response.

"Look," I told him, "I'm sorry, I'm going to call the chief or the surgeon because this is not good; we're wasting time," and I hung up.

Just as I got off the phone with the resident, the surgeon walked in.

"Lou," I said, "Look, this young guy's in liver failure. His liver has failed."

I presented all that data supporting this conclusion. I explained that he was going into a hepatic coma, becoming encephalopathic. He was filling up with poisons that his new transplanted liver was not able to detoxify. Because I had been a transplant nurse for over eight years, I determined this even without doing any neurological testing.

I was right. Indeed, his new blood work reflected a failed liver. The other critical liver lab values also reflected that fact. So did his urine. The brown dark sludge in his urine was bile that the liver was not utilizing properly (usually you excrete your bile in your stool, which is why your stool is brown). The fact that his labs were normal in the morning was meaningless because they had rapidly changed over the course of the shift.

"We have to put him back on the list to get a new liver," I told the surgeon. "We're wasting time by not being proactive."

The surgeon gave the patient a once-over and agreed that I was spot on. We immediately relisted the young man. He got a transplant, not that night but the next. Forty-eight hours later, he was sitting up in bed, eating, and chatting. Six days later, he went home with his parents and younger brother.

· · ·

Jo STECHER, PhD, MA, RN, CCTC, is a certified clinical transplant coordinator, was the Lung Transplant Coordinator at New York University Medical Center, and teaches at the School of Nursing at Florida Gulf Coast University in Fort Myers, Florida.

Hope in the Midst of Tragedy

Connie Barden

Years ago, before there was so much awareness about organ donation, the identification of patients as organ donors was much less automatic than it is today. Nurses were somewhat aware of the criteria used to identify an organ donor, but the systems in place to facilitate organ donation were more cumbersome and time consuming. At the same time, the need for donors was great, as it remains today.

I will never forget the experience of caring for a young man and his wife from Oklahoma who arrived in our intensive care unit. The couple had been on a cruise—celebrating their one-year anniversary—when the man suddenly collapsed. After being rescued and stabilized on the ship, he was airlifted to our hospital on a breathing machine and totally unresponsive to any stimulation. His CT scan showed that he had had a major hemorrhage in his brain, probably related to high blood pressure.

Over the next few days, the man progressed to being brain dead. The condition was explained to his wife, and she slowly absorbed that being "brain dead" meant that he was indeed dead even though his heart continued to beat and his chest continued to rise and fall because of the life support to which he was connected. The nursing staff mentioned organ donation to the physicians on the case one Friday morning, but the two doctors were not interested, stating that it would be "a lot of hassle" and that they thought it would be easier for the wife to just unplug the machines and let him go.

I had been involved in several similar situations in the twenty years of my career at that point and knew that for most families organ donation is a huge help in reckoning with the tragic and often premature loss of a loved one. A few of the nurses discussed the option, but because the physicians had opposed the idea they did not feel we should approach the family. My experience told me otherwise.

Nowadays, the organ procurement professionals do "the ask" for us, but in those days they did not. I sat with the wife and explained the phenomenon of brain death again. She told me about her husband and their short life together, including their hopes for children and dreams about the future. The young woman was devastated—far from home and with only one relative present for support.

Knowing the risk in going against what the physicians had stated, I made the decision to talk with her about organ donation anyway. I painstakingly explained the process and what it meant, outlined the potential good that such a young, healthy donor could bring, and gave examples of similar patients we had cared for who had become successful donors. Exhausted and overwhelmed, she asked for time to think about it. A little over an hour later, she paged me, and when I returned she told me she was ready to move forward with what it would take to have her husband become a donor. For the first time in four torturous days, I could see a flicker of peace and control in her face. She said to me, "Maybe at least something good can come out of this."

By this time it was after four on a Friday afternoon—not an optimal time to begin the process with our physician colleagues who had opposed the action from the start. After letting the surprised nursing staff know what I had done, I placed a call to the attending physician and neurologist to let them know the wife wished to proceed with donation. One physician—the neurologist—was annoyed and demanded to know how this had happened because he had not wanted to move in that direction and expressed his unhappiness that I had begun the process "on a Friday afternoon." I let him know that I had done it for the wife's well-being and because of her right to know about the option. I reminded him that there was absolutely no contraindication to the patient's being a donor and about the huge shortage of donors in this country. I let him know we would be calling the organ procurement agency very soon.

The surgery to remove the organs took place early that Saturday morning, and I came in to be with the wife until it was over. In the end, the patient was a fine donor and successfully donated several vital organs (kidneys, heart, liver) that were transplanted to multiple recipients—all of whom were facing imminent death.

For several years, I received notes and holiday cards from the wife from Oklahoma. Never did one of them arrive without containing her thanks for bringing up the organ donation option when she thought all her hopes for making peace with this tragic situation were gone. She reminded me that being offered that option was one of the things that helped to make it possible for her to recover from the tragedy and move on with her life.

• • •

CONNIE BARDEN, RN/CNS, MSN, CCRN, CCNS, is a Clinical Nurse Specialist in the electronic ICU, Baptist Health South Florida in Miami, and past president of the American Association of Critical Care Nurses.

The Advantages of Age

Marion Phipps

After forty years of being a nurse, my hair is white and my weight more than it should be. I sometimes wonder if this is due to the nature of the work of nursing, genetics, or, in the case of my weight, a too great love of food. On occasion, I find using my age and experience to be a useful tool to promote an aspect of patient care that I feel is important.

After working as a staff nurse for five years on a busy neurology unit I returned to graduate school. I have been a clinical nurse specialist since completing the program over thirty years ago. For the past seven years I have worked as a CNS on an acute neuroscience unit. Some days, I am a teacher, traffic cop, baseball coach, philosopher, and psychotherapist, all rolled into one often harried person. Taking deep, cleansing breaths is an essential and frequent activity.

One of our most difficult patient stories will stay with me forever. We had in our care a forty-eight-year-old woman I'll call Mrs. Smith, with a devastating fatal neurological disease that caused tumors in her brain stem and kidneys. Her husband and daughters, who adored her, believed she would recover and wanted her to live as long as possible. She had been hospitalized on our unit multiple times over a two-year period and continued to have neurological and functional decline. After a complicated and delicate surgery to remove more of the brain stem tumor, this woman was comatose and depended on a ventilator to breathe. Her condition was grave. She looked awful. She had lost over twenty pounds and appeared ashen and vulnerable. Her family continued to believe she would recover and wanted all measures, including cardiopulmonary resuscitation (CPR), performed.

The nursing staff talked a lot about this patient. Their great concern was that she would experience a cardiac arrest, and they feared having to perform CPR on such a fragile woman. They believed that performing chest compressions would lead to harm and have little impact on Mrs. Smith's outcome. Nursing staff began to dread being assigned to this woman's care because they knew her situation was so tenuous. They did not want to cause her any additional suffering. We talked a lot about the meaning of suffering and how it was expressed in Mrs. Smith's illness.

The neurosurgical resident caring for Mrs. Smith was one I respected. I felt he was a caring man who would become a fine doctor. We had talked often about other patients, and I felt we had a collaborative relationship. When I asked him if we could discuss this patient he sat down with me. However, when I described our worries about Mrs. Smith and asked for a palliative care consultation to support staff and the family, I was stunned by his response. He said no to the consultation: "I take care of her neck. Her neck is fixed, and that's where my job ends."

He walked away, leaving me sitting in a chair. I had been totally unprepared for his response, and I was upset and disappointed. I needed a few hours to recover. I wondered if he had been in the operating room all night and might have been exhausted. I reflected on what I tell our nurses all of the time: "You have such valuable information to give to the doctors. In many ways, we are teaching our young medical staff how to grow in their practice as we grow in ours."

I thought about this situation for a day and decided I needed to take a step toward this young physician. I sought him out as he was leaving the unit. I am a lot shorter than he; however, I reached up and put an arm on his shoulder. "Look at this gray hair of mine. I've been doing this work for a long time. I have been involved in the care of many patients as they approached their deaths. I'm near the end of my career, but you are just at the beginning of yours. I hope in the few years we will be working together I can influence you to consider that supporting patients at their end of lives is a really important part of your work as a neurosurgeon." He looked at me, blushed a little, and walked away. I was worried that I had gone a bit too far.

The next day he approached me on the unit and told me he had discussed a palliative care consultation with the attending surgeon and that he had placed an order that day.

Over the next few days I had several intense conversations with this woman's husband. He had met with the palliative care team and was reluctant to allow his wife to be made DNR (Do Not Resuscitate). One morning, after this woman had experienced nighttime unstable blood pressure and multiple cardiac arrhythmias, I approached the husband. I told him that the nursing staff feared having to resuscitate his wife. I asked him if he wanted to know what happened with resuscitation. He said he did. I told him as clearly as I could about the intensity of chest compressions, the possibility of fractured ribs in such a frail person, and our worry of causing his wife further suffering. He listened. He called his daughters. That day his wife was made DNR. The palliative care team instituted comfort care measures to keep her comfortable such as giving her medication to decrease her pulmonary secretions. A few days later, this woman died comfortably with her family at her side.

In our work, we must not forget the impact we can have on our colleagues and the patients and families in our care. Sometimes we have to take a risk and go in a direction that may not feel comfortable. Even after all of these years in nursing, I continue to learn and grow with each experience. And, in this situation, I used my white hair to my advantage.

• • •

Marion Phipps, RN, MS, CRRN, FAAN, has been a nurse for forty years. She is a clinical nurse specialist in neuro-rehabilitation.

An Expiration Date for Indignancy

Madeline Spiers

I was talking with nurses at the Irish Nurses Organization head-quarters in Dublin some years ago. They were attending an overseas nurses section, meeting mostly Filipino nurses. During coffee, Mary, a Filipino nurse with extensive experience nursing abroad, started chatting with me about working and living in Ireland. Here is one story she shared.

I work in the voluntary sector in an intellectual disability unit since I have come to Ireland. While I have a solid grasp of the English language now, it is often the cultural undercurrents that I do not understand. Some months ago I was caring for a fourteen-year-old boy with severe disabilities. He had a chest infection that required antibiotics, which were duly written up and ordered.

When the prescription arrived from the pharmacy, I checked the details, and the antibiotics were six months out of date. So I rang the pharmacy, explained the problem, and requested that they send new antibiotics. My patient was a very sick boy, and he needed the medicine to be in date and effective. The pharmacy rang back later and told me to use the antibiotics they had sent because they were "still all right."

I said, no, that expiration dates were there for a reason and it was against best practice.

Some time later, the unit manager arrived, and I explained the situation. Her response was, "Would you just give the antibiotics and avoid all the hassle?"

"The doctor has prescribed these drugs, which have to be in date to be effective, and I cannot fail my patient or my professional standards of care," I replied.

A little while passed before the house doctor (medical intern) rang the unit. His name was Dr. Paul. He was a busy young man. And very important. I knew immediately from his tone that the pharmacist and the manager had been in touch with him. "What is the problem?" he inquired.

I recounted the situation and waited for his response "Don't waste my time on this. Give the antibiotics to the patient."

"I would like to," I said, "but they are out of date."

There was a pause on the phone, and then he shouted, "I'm the doctor, and I'm telling you to give him the out-of-date antibiotics right now—*Do you hear me?*"

"I cannot do that," I said. "I cannot give medicine that is out of date."

With that, in a very strange voice, Dr. Paul said to me, "Who am I?" Then he repeated the same words, "WHO AM I?" shouting into the phone.

I became worried for him and said, "I know who you are, but if you don't know who you are then that is very worrying for you."

There was a long silence. The phone was put down and some time later new, correctly dated antibiotics arrived. Thankfully, my patient made a full recovery. That incident was never spoken about, and Dr. Paul seemed to remember who he was in the end. I have traveled far from home to work as a nurse to keep my family. I cannot lose my registration because of poor standards in some institutions. It is sometimes very hard to speak out, but when a person in your care is put at risk you just have to. My union protects me, and so I can protect my patients.

· · ·

MADELINE SPIERS, RGN, BA, M.Litt, was president of the Irish Nurses Organization 2004–2008 and president of the European Forum for Nursing and Midwifery Associations attached to WHO (2007–2009).

What Hospice Is For

Jean Chaisson

She was petite and forthright. "Do you think that I really need a nurse? I have been so fortunate in my life; isn't there a young mother without family to help her who needs your assistance more than I? Isn't there some poor young woman in Roxbury who's just had a baby and has no family that you could help instead?" Alice asked me.

I already knew Alice from a distance, having grown up in the same community. A tireless supporter of educational initiatives for inner-city children, low-income housing, and the League of Women Voters, she had spent decades putting her time, money, and voice into helping others. Now, after she had experienced some health problems, I was finally meeting her face to face as her home care nurse. She agreed to accept my assistance only after I had assured her that home care wasn't a zero-sum game and that both she and the poor young woman from Roxbury could receive care if they needed it.

Over a period of several weeks, I helped teach Alice about her health problems and her medications, and she stabilized on a regimen of anticoagulant medication, which would decrease her risk of having strokes. Her attending physician was a woman who had cared for Alice for many years. Alice was proud of her doctor and attached to her hospital, which she had visited many times. She was glad that women were now able to succeed in the field of medicine. Her doctor seemed to be fond of Alice, too, and was always quick to call me back when there were concerns or questions about Alice's health or medications. When Alice no longer met Medicare criteria for receiving routine home care, the doctor asked her to privately arrange to have me come in regularly to check her cardiac status and manage her medications.

As I visited Alice regularly over a period of years, her health steadily declined. Despite careful attention to blood pressure and medication, she had a number of small strokes. She slept most of the day, ate poorly, and was no longer able to easily get out of the home. Her family had hired live-in help to keep her safely cared for. But her doctor did not seem to realize how much Alice was slipping, often expressing frustration that Alice missed appointments, as if the problem was the inconvenience to the physician not the patient's failing health. When I let her know how rare it was for Alice to be up and ready to leave the house before four o'clock in the afternoon, her doctor seemed to be in denial, "She seemed fine when I saw her last!" I pointed out that Alice only got out on her very best days.

As Alice continued to decline, her family became more concerned about providing support for her. She now had trouble communicating her needs, was moved in a wheelchair, and had difficulty swallowing. She had been such a lively woman, and I was watching her disappear bit by bit. I discussed the possibility of hospice care with her sons and daughters, and they were excited about the promise of spiritual support for their mother, better control of the restlessness and agitation that sometimes unsettled the household, and the prospect of a peaceful death at home when the time came. They planned to ask about hospice at an upcoming visit with Alice's doctor. I expected the doctor to be responsive to this request and was, therefore, surprised to get a call from Alice's daughter the evening of the appointment. Both upset and astonished, her daughter reported, "Her doctor wouldn't agree to refer Mom to hospice. She doesn't feel that she needs it."

I put a call in to the doctor the next day. When she called me back, she sounded angry, focusing again on the difficulty that the family seemed to have getting Alice to keep appointments, and stating that Alice was not "right" for hospice because she did not have cancer. I patiently educated the doctor about the many reasons that people receive hospice care and articulated the reasons that Alice would qualify for this assistance. Her doctor was unmoved: "Well, I will not refer anyone for hospice unless they have cancer."

I called Alice's daughter, and let her know that I had not been able to obtain the doctor's permission for hospice care. All of Alice's children spoke to me over the next few days, reiterating their wish for hospice care and asking questions about their mother's health and prognosis. I told them that if they wanted hospice care for their mother, they would have to find a doctor who would be responsive to the patient's actual condition. This was hard for them to hear because of their mother's attachment to both doctor and hospital.

Finally Alice's daughter called me to let me know that they had made the difficult choice of changing physicians. They regretted disrupting the longstanding relationship that their mother had established with her doctor, but they trusted my judgment and knew that their mother needed and deserved hospice services.

Alice began seeing a new doctor, who didn't hesitate to agree to hospice care and worked closely with the hospice nurse and me. Because Alice and her family were attached to me, I continued to collaborate with hospice on her care. Alice died peacefully at home several months later.

. . .

JEAN CHAISSON, RN, MS, worked as a clinical nurse and a clinical nurse specialist in Boston-area hospitals for twenty years and now sees home care, hospice, and palliative care patients at home and in the hospital.

A Real Pain

Paola Scamperle

As a neurosurgical nurse I've got plenty to do, including helping patients with some of the things some doctors don't do well—one of which is effectively managing patients' pain. Let me give you an example. I recently took care of a patient whose surgeon insisted that he didn't need much nursing care. The patient had been operated on for a herniated disc and had only been out of surgery for one day. Interestingly, the patient himself was a senior physician, a gastroenterologist who'd come to our hospital and unit because of the spine surgeon's reputation.

As soon as I began to take care of him, the patient-physician asked me to tell him about the normal course of postoperative recovery for this kind of operation. I told him we usually discharged patients two days after their surgery and that we give them a prescription for pain medication. He was very concerned about pain meds because he'd been in unbearable pain before his surgery and took pain pills daily. After the operation he continued to take these pills but was still complaining about his pain. Plus, he had a lot of pain that we hadn't expected from the wound site.

When his well-respected surgeon came in to do a quick exam, the patient told him that he was in pain. Although this surgeon is very competent and self-confident, pain management is not one of his strengths. He just doesn't understand that pain is an exquisitely personal experience and that each patient experiences it differently.

So what was the doctor's response to this particular patient? He insisted the patient was somehow "imagining" his pain, not really having it. The surgeon told the patient that he'd checked on his surgery, all was well, and he should no longer be in pain. So even though I spoke with him about the patient's pain, he didn't come up with a different pain management strategy.

Not surprisingly, when it came time for his discharge two days later, the patient was still in so much pain that he couldn't leave the hospital. When the surgeon and a medical student made their rounds that day, the patient again asked them about his pain. Once again, they insisted that the patient's pain could not be as severe as he said it was.

By now, I'd been with the patient over several days. I watched how he walked and knew how uncomfortable he was. I knew I had to do something to manage his pain and recognized that ordinary pain-killers just wouldn't work.

The first thing I did was talk to the patient. In a careful tone, I said: "Look, Dr. X, your surgeon is very knowledgeable and competent. Most of the time patients don't have a lot of pain. But I know from experience that the kind of inflammatory pain you're having doesn't resolve within the first day or two. What you need is some cortisone prescribed in a single dose in the morning for a few days. I have seen this work in other cases with worse pain than yours."

The patient-physician thought about this. He thanked me for the suggestion and asked me to talk to the surgeon and suggest that he order the medication. I waited until the surgeon was out of the OR and talked with him. He'd become so frustrated with the patient that he quickly agreed. He ordered the medication, and I gave the cortisone to the patient. Pretty soon the patient was comfortable and appeared not only relaxed but serene. He approached me in the hall and said,

"I want to thank you so much for your patience, your availability, and most of all for your competence and the professional attitude you showed me these past days. If it hadn't been for you, I would still be in pain. I would have been suffering the same pain that made my life intolerable and led me to have this surgery in the first place. I want to thank you for dealing with this and all the needs I've had since I came to the hospital."

Nurses do these kinds of things everyday. Isn't it about time we advertised them?

· · ·

PAOLA SCAMPERLE, RN, works at Azienda Ospedaliera, Istituto Borgo Trento di Verona, Italy, in a neurosurgical unit, and has also worked in a general surgical ward and as a nursing instructor at the Ospedale Macchi di Varese and University of Insubria.

Part 4
NOT PART OF THE JOB DESCRIPTION

One of the enduring legacies of nursing's religious origins is the notion that nurses should be saintly creatures, always quick to sacrifice themselves for their patients. Of course, we should expect nurses to put aside their own personal needs when they're tending to a patient or during a crisis. (When a patient is in cardiac arrest, no nurse in the world leaves for a lunch break.) For the RN saint or angel, the expectation of self-sacrifice has no limits. Indeed, sometimes this self-sacrificing version of "professionalism" demands that nurses efface themselves entirely.

I've heard RN academics or managers tell students or staff nurses they shouldn't ask for a raise because they're supposed to be in it for love, not money. And I've watched nurses respond with, "we don't care about the money," as if they don't need to pay the rent or mortgage and put food on the table. I was once in a hospital where the call went out for nurses to volunteer to lift an eight-hundred-pound patient. The institution hadn't purchased lift equipment because it was sure RNs would rise to the occasion. Rather than fight to make sure the hospital had lift equipment, some did. Who knows how many people got hurt in the process? When an irate patient lashes out violently, nurses are supposed to consider the punch in the jaw or stomach an unavoidable part of the job.

Nurses report that they're routinely forced to skip lunch or coffee breaks. They sometimes can't even make it to the bathroom during an entire shift. They're also expected to navigate the hostile workplaces created by out-of-control medical colleagues or the high-risk patients that one sometimes meets in home care. When nurses finally ask to be treated like ordinary mortals, they're often made to feel like they're selfish or unreasonable. No wonder nurses adapt by boasting about how long they can hold it in, go without food, or otherwise tough it out in the workplace.

The problem is, saying yes to such demands produces demoralized, burnt-out nurses. More important, it produces nurses who suffer more back, neck, and shoulder injuries than stevedores or dock workers (who now press a button when they have to lift a crate); 6 to 11 percent of RNs leave the workplace due to such injuries each year. Because nurses are not disembodied angels, more RNs suffer from stress-related illnesses and depression than the rest of the population. In this case, the price of self-sacrifice is that the nurse now becomes a patient.

Given their socialization in self-sacrifice and the exploitative definitions of altruism they've learned, it's not easy for RNs to say no and to offer constructive alternatives to the status quo. That's why the stories of these RNs are so important and instructive. The nurses who recount their stories in this section have gone the extra mile for their patients many times. But they also insist on limiting the sacrifices that any nurse should be expected to make. They know that endless self-sacrifice doesn't help patients and can actually hurt them. Exhausted, burnt out, or injured nurses don't make good patient advocates. Which is why these nurses, and others, have rejected the idea that unsafe working conditions should be a standard part of anyone's job description.

I'll Call in Sick If I Have To

Barbara Egger

I was working in a long-term care facility when, one Saturday on the three-to-eleven shift, I walked in to discover I had three patients who had orders to use a Merry Walker (a safety device that reduces the risk of patients' falling and also protects nurses). Unfortunately, there were only two devices on the unit. I called the nursing office, explained the situation to my supervisor, and pleaded with her to find me another walker before someone fell and got hurt. She called me back, explaining that they were kept in a locked storage building out back. Then she told me the only employee with a key to the building did not work on weekends, so we would have to "make do" until Monday.

Sunday morning, before coming in to work, I called the supervisor's office and asked if they had gotten the needed equipment. When the answer was "no," I told the supervisor I was calling in sick because I had an awful knot in my stomach and not to expect me in for the evening shift.

On Monday, I was notified to report to see the director of nursing (DON) and hospital administrator. They asked me what I thought the board of nursing would think about a nurse who refused to work because she did not like the supplies available. I replied with the question, "What would the Department of Health say about a facility that wouldn't provide necessary safety equipment that was ordered for a patient because they didn't want to bother someone on a weekend?"

The floor got another Merry Walker that day, and I never heard another word about it.

• • •

BARBARA EGGER, RN, C BA, has been a nurse for over twenty-five years and comes from a family of nurses, including her grandmother, aunt, and five of her cousins, as well as her eldest daughter, an RN working on a pediatrics floor.

Doing the Heavy Lifting

Martha Baker

For way too long, hospitals have been asleep at the wheel when it comes to the kinds of musculoskeletal injuries that nurses suffer from and that jeopardize patient care. At Jackson Memorial Hospital and Health System in Miami, Florida, we decided to wake up our administrators by fighting for a safe lift program at the hospital as well as in the Florida state legislature.

There's a growing body of evidence that documents the problem of lifting in hospitals and other health care settings—much of it by Dr. Audrey Nelson, at the Veterans Administration in Tampa, Florida. This startling data shows that 18 percent of nurses leave the bedside each year because of a back or other kind of musculoskeletal injury. Another alarming fact is that 12 to 24 percent leave because of a perceived fear of such an injury. If you can eliminate these kinds of injuries and make the workplace safer, you can help to stem the nursing shortage in this country.

Making the workplace safer for nurses makes it safer for patients as well. Patient care also suffers because of improper lifting. In non–health care work settings—at a company such as UPS, for example—workers can get injured, and merchandise can be damaged. In health care, the stakes are higher. If a health care worker drops something, it won't be a cardboard box; it will be a vulnerable human being. Without teams that are educated about lifting and proper lift equipment, which is now readily available and pays for itself in only a matter of years, nurses or other health care workers can drop patients or otherwise seriously injure a patient. An elderly person who is dropped may suffer a hip fracture and even die. Or consider what happens when a nurse has no lift equipment or anyone to help her and has to drag a patient up in bed. The resulting skin shearing can cause skin breakdown that can cost between $25,000 to $75,000 based on the severity of the patient's injury.

Injuries to workers and patients can be prevented by a safe lift program. This means that no employee lifts more than fifty pounds. Whether it's a box delivered by UPS or a patient lifted by a nurse, we now know that no one—no matter how strong and burly—can safely lift more than fifty pounds without getting microfractures to the spine. Hospitals with a dedicated safe lift program mobilize a combination of lift equipment and appropriately trained staff to lift patients. So, if you have a three-hundred-pound patient, you'd need six people to lift that patient, or you could have a trained lift team that operates safe lift equipment. At Jackson, we decided to grapple with this issue by getting safe patient handling written into our contract with the hospital and approaching the issue legislatively. We took the legislative route because we believe that all two hundred hospitals in the state of Florida should have a safe lift program. We decided to fight for a lift team and lift equipment. Why? Because at Jackson, with its twelve thousand employees, having dedicated lift teams of twenty-five or so team members—who become experts on the equipment and help other employees to use it and to lift patients—means you don't have to train thousands of people in how to use lift equipment. This makes the program cost-effective.

In 2005, as we were negotiating our contract, we began to approach management as well as our nurses with the facts on the ground—the data about the costs: financial, physical, and emotional, of unsafe lifting. We demonstrated the savings a safe lift program can capture. Although there are direct costs of buying the equipment or hiring the team, savings are predicted to be four times the cost of the equipment and of educating a lift team or teams. There are savings on workers' compensation claims, on days lost if a nurse has an injury, and on replacement costs if a worker leaves the job permanently. And of course you're saving money—not to mention pain and suffering—if patients aren't injured.

As we negotiated with management, we not only marshaled the economic facts. On every possible occasion—Nurses' Week events, meetings around negotiations—we invited equipment vendors to bring their lift equipment into the hospital. Because Jackson is such a large hospital (3,600 nurses, 12,000 employees, and 2,400 beds systemwide), vendors were delighted to come and show off their wares.

We invited not only nurses but also upper management and even legislators to these events to see the equipment demonstrated. It was quite a sight to see employees and high-level administrators being hoisted up, swinging around the room, as vendors showed how effective and safe such equipment really is. As they say, a picture is—and indeed was—worth a thousand words.

It became clear to management that the concept of safe lifting was a winning proposition. Obviously, it's a lot better for patients to be lifted safely. The injuries to the nurses are reduced, which addresses the nursing shortage, not to mention physical harm to the employee. Finally, through a safe lift program, management wins financially. To us it was a no-brainer, but management initially resisted until we made a convincing economic case. And indeed, we won a safe lift program in the 2005 contract.

For us, that wasn't the end of the fight. The fact that we, at Jackson, have a safe lift program doesn't help workers and patients at the other 199 hospitals in Florida. Which is why we are persisting in our effort to legislate safe lift programs in all Florida hospitals. In 2008, the bill failed. But we will keep trying until it finally passes and protects us all.

• • •

MARTHA BAKER, RN, BSN, is Nurse Manager of the Trauma Intensive Care Unit at Florida's Jackson Memorial Hospital, president of Florida's SEIU Local 1991, a national leader of the SEIU Nurse Alliance, and chair of the National Workplace Quality Committee.

Attacked by a Patient, Abandoned by My Hospital

Charlene L. Richardson

In March 2003, I was working in the emergency room at Beverly Hospital, in Beverly, Massachusetts, when I was attacked by a patient. I was trying to discharge the patient, who had been in the ER all day. Although we were having difficulty getting him a ride, I am still not sure why he became so agitated. But suddenly, he brutally and viciously attacked me.

I was on the phone trying to get him a ride, and as I was hanging up, he lunged forward and grabbed me between the legs. Then, still hanging on to me, he stood up. He was a very big guy—and he wouldn't let go.

We were in a private room, and, although a fellow nurse was near, I knew I would be in terrible trouble if no one who could assist me against my assailant saw what was happening. So I backed myself into the hallway where, I hoped, someone could see what was going on and help. Another nurse witnessed this, ran over, and tried to free me from his grasp. Nothing she did could free me. His grip was so tight I could feel that he'd ripped through my uniform. The harder we worked to stop the assault, the tighter he held on, and I could feel with the area of my body that he was gripping tighter by the second that I was getting injured, as the pain was excruciating. By that time it felt like it was going in slow motion and taking forever, even though it was happening so quickly.

Although I tried to free myself when he first attacked me, I was still in you-don't-want-to-hurt-the-patient mode. As nurses it is always our intention to do no harm, and sadly our commitment to patient care leaves us very vulnerable to such attacks, especially when working on the front line that emergency nursing is. As it became clear that he was becoming increasingly aggressive and that no one could get him off of me, I somehow managed to wrest free of the hold he had between my legs. As soon as I did that, he grabbed on to the Kelly clamps that I had attached to my uniform (a lot of ER nurses carry them because if, god forbid, you have to deliver a baby quickly, or need them for any urgent reason you have a pair of clamps on you). He used the clamps quite differently—he tried to drive them through my leg.

At that point I realized that I was going to be seriously harmed if not killed. I remember what was going through my head, my being married to a police officer at that time: Oh my god, I am here to "do good" and I am fighting for my life. I had to free myself. Multiple people witnessed this event and although several came to my rescue, because of his size and determination to do harm, we were unsuccessful at getting me free. I remember also thinking to myself, at that point an eleven-year veteran nurse, I am not going to allow myself to be killed or maimed by this aggressive person.

With my street smarts and training in protecting myself against aggressive behavior, I was finally able to get free from his tight grasp, get him to the floor, and restrain him. But sadly, we became more entangled, and he landed on my leg. He had these big work boots on and although I didn't even realize it until I got home that night, I had a broken toe and he had completely ripped the toenail off inside my shoe.

The police came in and arrested him. Although I was in shock, I filled out the police reports and pressed full charges against him. I filled out an incident report and an employee accident report. Since there was no in-house supervisor I notified my nurse manager of the event. The evening of this awful event I was working as the charge nurse and the Emergency Room was on overload with high census and with very sick patients. So, as nurses do, I brushed myself off, went back to work, and then went home in shock. We are so used to taking care of others we forget about ourselves. We live in the moment and as nurses we think and act for the "greater good" at the sacrifice of ourselves. I didn't fully realize for a long, long time how deeply affected I was by the assault. But what was more upsetting was how my hospital responded to what happened.

In the judicial system, it can be a lengthy process to get a court date. It was four months before I received notification of the pretrial conference hearing. It was at this point I noted that the incident and employee accident reports I had filled out were nonexistent and had disappeared. Summonses were sent to the hospital to the witnesses of the assault yet were never received. This included the security guards who had responded the night of the assault. I notified my employer of my concern as the trial was approaching and let them know I fully intended on pursuing the charges against my assailant.

When I finally did pursue charges, I was met by complete resistance by my employer. My witnesses scheduled to testify were notified by the hospital that they could attend the trial but would not be paid. Even though the assailant had a long criminal record, the hospital did not back me up.

As a nurse, I was committed to safe patient care and gave 150 percent; the worst thing possible happened to me on the job while I was giving that 150 percent. But my employer gave me less than nothing in return. Not only did my employer not give me support, I was never offered any type of debriefing after the attack, nor did a single administrator ever call me to ask if I was okay.

I was asked not to pursue charges against my attacker. The hospital was concerned about bad publicity, and because of the severity of the attack and the assailant's determination to stay out of prison, it was watched closely by the media. This was because he would plead guilty the day of the trial and then at the last minute before being sentenced he would rescind his plea and a new trial date would have to be scheduled. It took nearly eighteen months to prosecute the assailant and he received the maximum sentence allowed in the Commonwealth for this type of crime, eighteen months.

Because I had continued to pursue the charges, I went from ER Nurse of the Year and an exemplary employee to a problem employee. The administration of my hospital tried to wrongfully discipline me. It was at this point I realized my spirit was broken and felt as though my soul had been taken from me. I notified the Massachusetts Nurses Association (MNA), our union, which had to intervene on my behalf in a number of instances. I received assistance from the workplace violence taskforce, and the union intervened when the hospital attempted to quiet me on speaking about the attack. I was labeled a troublemaker and told that I was creating a hostile environment. My charts and documentation were closely scrutinized by administration, and I nearly suffered disciplinary action when I called the police for assistance during multiple instances of violence against employees.

I realized that I had to fight not only for myself but for other nurses who have too long been told that accepting violence in the workplace is a part of our job description. I knew at this point that emotionally I was very injured, and I wanted to ensure that no nurse would endure such injury and suffer the way I did. This fight led me to lobby, along with the MNA and other nurses, for legislation that would change current Massachusetts law. Right now, we have a law that protects emergency medical technicians, firefighters, and prehospital workers, e.g. ambulance workers, against assault. Under this law, if a police officer arrives at the scene after the incident takes place but doesn't witness the assault, an arrest can be made.

But everything changes when a patient crosses the threshold and enters the hospital. If that patient lays a hand on anybody in the hospital and the police don't witness it, the patient can't be arrested at that time. It is considered a past assault and unless witnessed by a police officer, no arrest can be made. The hospital worker has to press charges against the patient after the fact. (In my case, an arrest was made after the fact because a sexual assault is considered a felony.) This is why we're fighting to add nurses and other hospital workers to a law that already protects other workers.

It's not a lot to ask. This legislation is really a no brainer so I don't understand why we can't get it out of committee. I have continued to pursue this because I have suffered such loss and have been so injured by this incident. I left the Emergency Room after my assailant was prosecuted and sent to prison to allow myself to heal, vowing never to return to an Emergency Room to work again. During that time I have worked in the Recovery Room and then for the Massachusetts Nurses Association as Associate Director in both government legislation and nursing education. Just over three years ago, after intense therapy, I returned to the Emergency Room and now work on a per diem basis. I also obtained my certification in Legal Nursing and have nearly completed my Masters Degree in Nursing. I've been working on this since my attack, and I'm not going to stop until we are all protected.

• • •

CHARLENE L. RICHARDSON, BSN, RN, CEN, LNC, was Associate Director of Government and Legislation and is now Associate Director of Nursing Education at the MNA. An RN for nearly nineteen years, she has a specialty in recovery post anesthesia nursing, is a board certified Emergency Room Nurse, and is also a Legal Nurse Consultant. She received the Political Organizer Activist award from the North Shore Labor Council and AFL-CIO in 2008.

The Samurai Sword

Anne Duffy

As the leader of a union that represents ten thousand home care nurses in the United Kingdom, my job is to make sure that our nurses are safe. They work in inner cities, as well as in other dangerous and remote areas. When they knock on the door of a patient's home, they never know whom or what they're going to find behind that door. Some of our nurses have experienced terrible verbal and physical abuse. So we're constantly surveying our members to get data on the problem of violence in the workplace—which in this case is the patient's home. With that data we go back to our government representatives, in this case health ministers, to ask for money to make nurses' work safer.

To fight for nurses, however, I often find myself having to challenge nurses who have been socialized to accept the idea that they have to put up with violence in their workplace, that it's part of the job description.

A couple of months ago, I went to an area of Liverpool, a city in northern England with high unemployment, to try to find out about incidents of violence toward nurses in patients' homes. I visit cities all over the United Kingdom to meet with nurses and hear their concerns as violence against National Health Service workers is on the increase, and I knew that nurses here come across abuse on a daily basis and they are often reluctant to report these incidents to management. I always need up-to-date statistics in order to make a good case for funding for nurse safety to health ministers. I had an upcoming appointment to meet with the Prime Minister, Gordon Brown, and wanted to raise this issue with him.

While I was talking to a group of nurse members in Liverpool, I asked if they'd ever been assaulted or abused in the workplace.

"No, no," they said, "we can't think of any time we've been assaulted."

I was standing there with two of my professional officers and thinking, this is all wrong. I know people are getting attacked up here; I had talked with other nurses on the telephone who were off work following physical attacks by patients.

One of the guys who was with me started asking more probing questions. "So none of you has ever had a patient or patient's relative block your entrance or exit?" he asked.

"Oh yeah, of course; that happens all the time," they replied.

"Has anybody ever pushed or shoved you?" he continued.

"Oh yeah, that happens all the time," they said.

Then one nurse chimed in, "Well, recently, I had a guy pull a samurai sword on me and put it at my throat."

Shocked, I asked her if she'd reported it, and she said, no, she didn't think it was worth reporting.

I was utterly dismayed. Taking a deep, deep breath, I asked, "So have I got this right? Another nurse was going to see this same man the next day, and you didn't think any of your colleagues needed to be warned that this guy is extremely dangerous?"

"Oh, I didn't see it that way," she said. "I didn't think of that. I was just so glad to get out of the house because the samurai sword was so close to my throat."

During this meeting and many others, we kept trying to reinforce the message that anything that makes them uncomfortable needs to be reported. They need to do this because management records all the incidents and feeds them all the way up to the government.

Believe me, we did not let the samurai sword incident go unmentioned. I used it when I spoke to our Congress, and journalists reported on it. And believe me Gordon Brown PM also knows about it. In 2008, I was appointed to represent our union on the Security Implementation Group at the Department of Health in Whitehall, a working group of very senior health service managers, trade union leaders, and senior civil servants appointed by the current government to research the security and protection of staff while in the workplace.

As a result of our efforts, the Labour Government promised the National Health Service sixty-seven million pounds to be invested in safety for health care workers.

. . .

ANNE DUFFY has worked as a nurse and nurse manager in northern Ireland, Dublin, and England and as a professional advisor and researcher in Sweden, Italy, and Ethiopia. She is currently CEO of the Community and District Nurses Association in the U.K. and a nurse advisor on a project training Ethiopian nurses with the global charity Children in Crossfire.

Only When It's Safe

Bernie Gerard

It was a typical Saturday morning at my hospital. In other words, busy as hell. It was also my third week of orientation at my new job. I had been an RN for only eight months. I was working in a major trauma and surgical intensive care unit (STICU) at the University of Medicine and Dentistry in New Jersey, and boy, did I understand that I wasn't ready to fly on my own.

The call came in at 7:30 a.m., one half-hour into the shift: "Send Gerard to the coronary care unit." I could not believe what I was hearing.

"I can't go!" I practically screamed. "I'm still on orientation here. How do you expect me to function on a unit I know nothing about?"

The charge nurse told me that I had to go.

"I can't; *it's not safe,*" I insisted.

Word went out to administration, and at 8:30 a.m. I was called into the nursing lounge to be confronted by an angry and threatening nurse supervisor, a nurse director of surgical services, and the charge nurse from my unit. The three of them surrounded me, the new grad.

The first words from the nurse supervisor were, "Mr. Gerard, what's this I hear that you are refusing to go to CCU!"

I told her that I did not refuse to go. I explained that I was concerned for my patients' safety. I had not completed the three-month orientation in my own unit, I barely knew where supplies were kept, and I had a preceptor with me the entire time. Putting me in a strange unit could jeopardize patient care. I didn't know the protocols, doctor contact procedure, and so on, and I had a hard enough time functioning safely on my own unit. How could I, a novice, function safely in a totally unfamiliar setting? I asked.

The supervisor seemed to soften a bit. Nonetheless, with an edge to her voice, she asked, "So, you are not refusing to go to CCU?"

"No, definitely not. I never refused to go. I am just worried about finding my way around the unit so that I can function effectively and safely."

The supervisor looked at her director of service and asked if an orientation could be arranged and someone made available to help me in the CCU.

Yes, the director said, this could be arranged. So they all agreed that I would go to the CCU that day after I reported off on my patients in the STICU.

When I arrived on the CCU, the supervisor was there along with the charge nurse for the unit and the nurse assigned to orient and help me for the day. We exchanged pleasantries and introductions, and I was oriented to my "new unit." My day went well, without further incident.

What do you suppose it could have been like if I had not taken a stand that day? I know I was only able to give safe care that day because I spoke up.

Four years later, thanks to the efforts of the new union we had just organized at the hospital, defined orientation programs are in place as well as prohibitions on floating nurses from units in the hospital where they have experience to units where they have none.

• • •

BERNIE GERARD, RN, is First Vice President Health Professionals and Allied Employees (AFT, AFL-CIO), New Jersey.

The Red Shirts Are Coming

Mary Crabtree Tonges

As a chief nurse executive, I occasionally find myself standing up for nurses by stealth. For example, I was working for a large organization that had just undergone a work and job redesign initiative, popular in the late 1980s through the early 1990s, in which nursing assistants (NAs) learned to draw blood, take electrocardiograms (EKGs), and perform other skills that do not require licensure. They could function as multiskilled workers, Clinical Services Technicians (CSTs). This change made phlebotomy and EKG more readily available on the unit and decreased potential stand-by time for unlicensed clinical staff waiting for further direction from a nurse.

The project was successful and popular, resulting in the widespread conversion of NA positions to jobs for CSTs. To help patients identify caregivers in their different roles and present a professional appearance, nursing leaders decided that CSTs would wear a red top and white slacks as their uniform on all the units.

Those of us in the nursing division were happy with the change. Staff nurses appreciated the additional assistance with tasks, CSTs enjoyed the career progress and chance to practice new skills, and nursing leadership had a more productive role and a consistent dress code for these staff members.

Unfortunately, I began to hear less than positive comments from peers in administration—for example, half-joking remarks from finance and operations executives about seeing "all those red shirts" around the hospital or taking up spaces in the parking facilities. The innuendo was that nursing was overstaffed, never a good thing to be rumored. What to do? Respond to the negative peer pressure and reduce the number of CSTs, or ignore the comments in the hope that they would stop?

Because we were not overstaffed, I most definitely did not want to freeze or cut positions. Nonetheless I was getting rather tired and, more important, concerned about the not-so-funny "jokes" I kept hearing. These types of remarks are often an early warning about what's on people's minds, which may indicate a problem just around the bend and coming down the road. I decided I could easily solve the perceived problem by asking each clinical service to choose a different colored top, such as blue for cardiac, green for surgery, and so on. That way no one would see so many red shirts anymore.

Interestingly, this change in uniforms actually gave the CSTs more feelings of pride and association with their specialty area, what's widely known as a "win-win." Nothing changed but the color of the shirt, staffing was stable, the remarks stopped, and the CSTs, staff nurses, and nurse leaders were still happy.

I'm reminded of a story a CEO told me about a seemingly intractable problem he had while responsible for food service. Patients were dissatisfied with his roast beef despite new conveyor belts, warming carts, and multiple other interventions . . . until he changed the name to "pot roast."

· · ·

Mary Crabtree Tonges, RN, PhD, is Senior Vice President and Chief Nursing Officer, University of North Carolina Hospitals and Associate Dean for UNC Health Care in the School of Nursing, Chapel Hill, NC.

Not Saints or Sisters

Belinda Morieson

I've been a nurse for almost forty years and have watched nursing in Australia evolve from the English tradition with its background of church and army, when nurses wore veils and were called "sister." They went "on" and "off duty" and were infused with a sense of obligation and the need to always act with decorum. Unquestioning obedience was expected, as were poor pay and working conditions.

In the late 1970s I was working full time in Melbourne, raising three children, and enrolled part time in a university arts degree program. Like so many other nurses, I understood the rules and abided by the work ethic and accepted poor pay. But as I grew older and had the expense of raising children, I also started meeting people who earned twice as much as I did and who had a great deal less responsibility. Furthermore they didn't do shift work. I began to realize that in addition to being underpaid, my goodwill was being abused. It was said that nursing was a "vocation," thus excusing the government from paying us the appropriate salaries and giving us the professional respect given to other health professionals. Like some other nurses, I finally got annoyed.

I would hear nurses say "I am just a nurse," and I thought how wrong we are not to shout from the rooftops "I am a nurse: I am intelligent, hard working, educated, and care for the most vulnerable in the community."

In 1982 I became a union workplace rep in the Victorian Branch of the Australian Nursing Federation (ANF), one of two union reps in the metropolitan hospital where I worked with over two thousand nurses. In 1984 I became a charge nurse; by then, with a lot of time and effort, I had increased the number of union reps to twelve. Together we raised the profile of the union in that hospital. We had several disputes with management, all successfully resolved in our favor through negotiation.

In 1986 I was seconded into the union to work on a new career structure and talk to management across the state about its implementation.

The hospital managers were genuine in their intention to implement the career structure, but the government refused to provide
funding. The government at the time was Labour, and in my experience neither Labour nor Conservative governments are willing to
adequately fund nursing, and the only way to achieve proper funding is by forcing them to do so by industrial action and by playing on
the fact that the community will always support nurses before politicians. So we shed our "decorum" and went on strike for fifty days to
achieve an appropriate career structure and salary.

Although this lengthy strike was successful, many nurses suffered
both emotionally and financially. During the next few years, we developed a new tactic that we used when we bargained our contracts
with the government for the public health system in Victoria, which
covers approximately 70 percent of our hospital beds and provides
high-quality care free of charge.

Instead of going on strike, nurses would close beds and operating
room (OR) sessions across the state. If a unit had twenty beds, we'd
agree to take care of patients in sixteen of them, but not in the other
four. There were exceptions—obstetrics, pediatrics, oncology, intensive care, cardiac critical care unit, and any emergency admissions.
But there were no elective admissions. By doing this, we won our
strike.

The first time we did this, we had no support from doctors, who
would try any means to get their elective admissions into a closed
bed. To be effective, the nurses had to hide the mattresses. Over time
the attitude of doctors changed, and they now offer support. Today,
nurses need only to put a notice on the bed to indicate that it is
closed. During the period that the industrial bans are in place, each
hospital forms a committee with doctors, nursing management, and
union reps as members. They meet each day to jointly determine
which patients will be admitted.

In 1999, when I was secretary of the Victorian Branch of the Australian Nursing Federation, we had to use bed closures to win one
of the most important patient care and nursing advances in the his-

tory of our union—even in the history of our country and the rest of the world. For over a decade, our country's most conservative government—led by Premier Jeff Kennett—had cut funds to the public health system and eliminated three thousand nursing positions. Nurses were overworked, and patient care eroded. By 1999, the citizens of Victoria as well as its nurses had had enough. They got rid of the Kennett government and elected a new Labour government, led by Steve Bracks.

By 1999, nurses were also fed up with working conditions in Victorian hospitals. Nurses were working long hours, struggling for resources, and finding they were constantly unable to have the time or support to deliver the kind of quality care they had gone into nursing to provide. They were burnt out and getting out fast because nursing was no longer the career they thought it would be. The ANF anticipated that, if this crisis were not addressed immediately, within five years there would be few permanent nurses working in Victoria's health system. As we entered bargaining, we heard about the nurse-to-patient ratios that had just been legislated in California and decided, in our bargaining claim, to demand a variety of different safe nurse-to-patient ratios in all public-sector hospitals.

We made the proposal, and the government said no. We had no choice but to initiate bed closures. We began the bans by closing one in six beds and one in six OR sessions across the state public health system. We also took our case to the public, which was concerned about deteriorating care in the public-sector hospitals on which it depended and supported us when we explained we would ensure that every patient got the care they needed.

When we went back to the negotiating table, the government wouldn't budge and neither would the nurses. The nurses increased the bans to close one in five beds and OR sessions, then one in four. It was when we threatened to close more beds that the government took the dispute to the Australian Industrial Relations Commission (AIRC)—a national body that arbitrates industrial disputes—for resolution.

By this time, it was the year 2000. We'd moved into the next century, but the government wanted us to continue as if we were still in the last one. Moreover, the AIRC and the government ordered me to direct the nurses to open the beds. I refused. I was then threatened with being taken to federal court, where refusal to obey a directive could result in being sent to jail. "So send me to jail," I replied. "I will not direct the nurses to open the beds until the government makes a satisfactory offer that is acceptable to the nurses."

As I heard myself saying this, I was as surprised as the government representatives I was talking to. "What the hell am I saying?" I wondered. Sure, I usually enjoy new experiences, but becoming a prisoner was not one of them. I had to believe that the government wouldn't be foolish enough to jail the leader of the nurses' union—a person who had the support not only of the nurses she represented (some of whom wrote me e-mails saying they'd go to jail in my place) but also of a public that highly regards nurses. I even got letters of support from blue-collar male unions, whose leaders offered to support us during our actions.

After we presented our case to AIRC Commissioner Wayne Blair, who was hearing the disputing parties, on August 31, 2000, Blair decided in favor of the nurses. We won one-to-four nurse-to-patient ratios (plus a charge nurse with no patient assignment) on medical-surgical floors, and specified ratios on other units depending on the relative acuity of patients. The government was furious. But it was Blair's decision that awarded the ratios. And the government had to abide by it. Because the government was forced into this, they then spent heaps of money in running reentry programs for people who'd been out of nursing for a long time. They did an enormous amount of advertising in state as well as interstate. We gave them additional time to reduce the agency nurses. Since the agency nurses could no longer get the work through agencies many of them then joined on as permanent staff.

Because we acted forcefully and argued from the facts on the ground, Blair gave us an outstanding deal. We got back so much we'd lost. We increased the nursing workforce by over three thousand in a short time and a lot of them came from interstate and reentry programs. Besides the safer nurse-to-patient ratios, we also got additional nurse educators, additional senior nurse clinicians, a qualification allowance if you went back to university and got additional credentials, additional night duty allowance, paid study leave, and seminar leave. We nurses had stood up for ourselves and our patients, and we won.

· · ·

BELINDA MORIESON, RN, is past Secretary of the Australian Nursing Federation, Victorian Branch.

Part 5

WHEN ONE ADVOCATE CAN MAKE A DIFFERENCE

In nursing school and on the job, nurses are expected to be, and think of themselves as, patient advocates. But what does advocacy really involve? The word itself comes from the Latin verb *vocare*—which means "to call." In this case, however, it doesn't refer to a vocational calling (as in nursing or the priesthood). As Webster's defines the term, an *advocate* is "one who pleads in a court of law, who defends a cause by argument." To defend patients today, RN advocacy almost always requires some sort of public calling out of those in power.

Nurses take great pride in being patient advocates. Many consider themselves to be the only ones in the health care system who fight for and protect patients. This creates a lot of dissension among other professionals and groups of health care workers who also consider themselves to be both caring and concerned about patients' well-being. As one physician put it when he heard a nurse explain that she was the patient's advocate: "What does that make me, the patient's enemy?" I've even heard social workers express their distress that nursing was trying to hijack the notion of patient advocacy. One told me, "Sometimes I think the first thing students learn in nursing school is that RNs are the only ones who care about patients and that they have to protect their patients from everyone else in the system."

The irony of nurses' claim that advocacy is their exclusive property is that many times the concept of advocacy is misunderstood. Again, advocacy requires some sort of public stance, argument, or expression of intent. Even if that advocacy is expressed in what seems like a private conversation between a doctor and a nurse, that act of advocacy is "public"—it takes place outside the head of the individual nurse. Some nurses, however, insist they are patient advocates even if they shy away from any public expression or risk that advocacy involves: If you wish the patient well, hope they do well, and have good, kind thoughts about the patient, then that's enough. But just having kind thoughts about a patient isn't real advocacy. It's the chicken soup that isn't enough.

In these stories of individual advocacy, we see real advocacy in action. The RNs involved sometimes risked their jobs and careers. While the stakes were high, they succeeded in making changes that improved the health and well-being of both individuals and entire populations, ranging from students in a public school system to elderly and infirm patients living on their own in remote areas. Their forceful intervention affected the way that doctors or health care administrators dealt with long-neglected problems. Their courage and persistence transformed the way that policymakers and politicians view the role of nurses.

Putting Lymphedema on the Map

Saskia R. J. Thiadens

It was 1983. I was running a postoperative care facility in San Francisco for patients to recuperate after cosmetic and reconstructive postcancer surgery. On this day, I picked up a patient from the University of California, San Francisco recovery room. She had undergone breast reconstruction following breast cancer surgery. I noted her huge swollen arm and became alarmed, thinking that it could be an allergic reaction. I called her surgeon immediately and remember that he was annoyed with me for calling him about this, intimating that I was stupid.

"At least, tell me what it is and how to treat it?" I asked him.

He could not give me a straight answer, nor did he know the name of the condition and was obviously in a rush to end our conversation. He finished our call by telling me that the patient had had this problem for nine years, and there was no treatment for this condition; she had learned to live with it.

I certainly did not accept this; nobody can live with an arm that size—not able to pick up grocery bags or her grandchildren or do a multitude of other daily tasks. I was both puzzled and frustrated. Since I wanted to help her, I immediately started looking for answers, initially by contacting some of the doctors I worked with at the time. For the first time, I heard the word *lymphedema* and was told that this condition—characterized by localized fluid retention and tissue swelling—can develop after breast cancer surgery when lymph nodes are removed from the armpit.

My next question was, is there a treatment, and can I help this unfortunate patient? At the same time, I was eager to learn more about the disease—its underlying cause, treatment, prevention, and genetic implications.

Shortly thereafter, I found that there was a clinic in the Black Forest in Germany where they were treating patients with lymphedema

107

through manual lymph drainage and a specialized bandaging technique. Moreover, I discovered that there were hundreds of thousands of patients, young and old, male and female and even newborns, affected by this condition worldwide. At that point, I knew I had to do something.

I closed the postoperative care facility and decided to start a clinic that would be primarily for patients with lymphedema. I rented space in a large medical building, occupied mostly with doctors' offices, and soon opened the first lymphedema clinic in the United States. Quickly the word spread that there was a nurse in San Francisco who helped patients with swollen limbs, and the phone rang off the hook. In no time, patients were in line outside my office pleading for answers and help.

In the meantime, the physicians in my building were not happy that a nurse had moved in and would turn their heads the other way when passing me in the hallway. What did I do wrong? I asked myself. I was trying to help underdiagnosed patients with a disabling condition and did not understand why these doctors viewed my actions so negatively. Well, it did not take much time for me to figure it out. The physicians were anxious about a nurse starting a clinic and questioning how I was able to bring all these patients to my office.

Soon the physicians began to ask me out for lunch to pick my brain about lymphedema. After a couple of months, I was overwhelmed with the number of patients and became aware of the enormity of this disease. At that time I had to make a decision: either close my doors or start a national clearinghouse to educate patients, professionals, and the general public about lymphedema.

In March 1988, I founded the National Lymphedema Network (NLN), a nonprofit organization, and ran it out of the clinic. At the helm of this new organization, however, I was twice as overwhelmed and busy because I was working double-duty: treating patients on a daily basis and reaching out to the local and national medical community, patients, and the general public through the NLN. It was a tough period in my life. In January 1989, I published the first issue of *Lymphlink,* the official NLN newsletter, sending it to breast cancer centers, hospitals, doctors' offices, and support groups.

In response to the newsletter mailing, a physical therapist and a doctor from Chicago called to tell me they were thrilled that I had founded the NLN and wanted to join forces with me. Getting this call from the doctor was quite a turnaround from my prior experience. In the clinic's early days, many doctors would not confess their lack of knowledge about lymphedema, particularly that they didn't even know what it was. They had to admit that a nurse knew more about this medical condition if they were to become educated in treatment and referral. I vividly remember a physician from Stanford University asking to visit my clinic. When he observed the manual lymphatic drainage procedure, he laughed and said this was a voodoo treatment and told the patient that this nurse was just taking her money.

One of the main reasons that lymphedema has been ignored until recently is that the lymphatic system is not part of the medical school curricula, and most physicians have no knowledge of—nor even an interest in—it. However, over the last twenty years, we have succeeded in putting lymphedema and the lymphatic system on the map. Through the determination of a handful of my patients, who knocked at doctors' office doors and encouraged patients to start support groups, we could begin to help the thousands of patients who are affected by this lifelong chronic condition.

Once I began successfully treating patients with lymphedema, I had to tackle the reimbursement problem. It was a battle because insurance companies did not recognize the diagnosis or did not consider the treatment medically necessary. I used the preauthorization request letters as an educational and awareness process. I wrote detailed letters to physicians and insurance companies alike and provided explicit information about what lymphedema is, its cause, how to treat it, and the benefits of treatment. It was important to highlight how cost-effective treatment was because lymphedema is a chronic condition and requires treatment plus wearing compression garments for the rest of the person's life.

One day, a patient came to see me with her son. She told me that her arm had doubled in size in the last few days and expressed great concern and discomfort. Her son told me that they saw the surgeon, and he told her that there was nothing he could do for her but not to worry.

It was obvious to me that she likely had a recurrent tumor that was blocking the lymphatics in her arm and causing the swelling. I am not a medical doctor but a nurse who received my degree from The University of Utrecht in Holland; however, I felt it was necessary to tell the son of this probable diagnosis. A few days later, I received a call from the patient's angry surgeon, yelling at me: "How dare you tell my patient that she has recurrent cancer?" I told him I had no choice but to do so. A couple months passed, and I was asked to do grand rounds for surgeons at a local hospital. I shared images of patients with upper- and lower extremity lymphedema, including cases of sudden increase in swelling, which usually indicates recurrent cancer. While I talked, I saw the surgeon who scolded me sitting in the front row. At the end of my talk, I asked if there were questions, and he raised his hand. My blood pressure started to rise. Rather than asking a question, he blushed, then thanked me and told his colleagues that "sometimes nurses are right." Moreover, he admitted his misdiagnosis.

Over the years, physicians in the San Francisco Bay area began to respect me, consult with me, and ask me for advice about their patients' swollen limb. Lymphedema had finally come to the medical forefront in the United States.

In the meantime, I needed to learn if professionals were treating and helping patients outside this country. I heard about and decided to attend the International Society of Lymphology (ISL) Conference in Tokyo in 1989. This, too, was an eye-opener. Clearly, these were the "old boys'" clubs, researchers from around the world who spend many hours a day focusing and often arguing the basic science of the lymph system, while my immediate interest was how we can treat and help our patients.

I soon became aware that I was the only clinician at this meeting and saddened by their treatment of me: instead of including me in discussion and drawing on my years of clinical experience, I was ignored when asking a question and identified as that "stupid blond nurse." Later, I learned that one of the doctors thought I came to the meeting to find a husband! Twenty years later, the roles have reversed: Many of the ISL physicians now ask me to speak at their meetings or insist that they be invited to attend or lecture at the NLN Biennial International Conferences I organize.

Since the founding of the NLN, we have moved into mainstream medicine with thousands of professionals becoming certified lymphedema therapists through specialized training courses; physicians are beginning to add the lymphatic system into their existing practices; the NLN "position papers" are being widely used in affiliated NLN clinics, hospitals, breast centers, doctors' offices, and cancer support groups; and basic and clinical research and trials are actively done in academic institutions around the country.

NLN distributes a thirty-six-page newsletter, *LymphLink*, to over three thousand members and has organized eight successful international conferences bringing together experts from around the world.

Most important, patients with lymphedema now are receiving the care they require and deserve.

· · ·

SASKIA R. J. THIADENS, RN, has worked in numerous nursing capacities and founded the National Lymphedema Network (NLN) in 1988, where she is still at the helm as the executive director.

An Inconvenient Nurse

Faith Henson

I became a nurse at the age of fifty-five, fulfilling a life-long dream. I accepted a job in a local hospital, full of idealism, commitment, and a love of nursing. At that time I would never have envisioned the path that lay ahead, the obstacles I would have to overcome, or the positive changes in my commitment to nursing and personal strength.

Since then, over the past ten years, I have managed to get myself fired for being a vocal patient advocate, a union organizer, and a whistleblower. As is often true, each time it was a blessing in disguise, as another more challenging door opened. I have never regretted anything I have done or said, and know that I implemented many changes in health care that have been beneficial to patients. This story is about the thing I am most proud of, which resulted in a significant change in health care and has spread nationwide.

The first four years of my RN career, I worked happily at the small hospital in my hometown. Gradually, I felt more comfortable with my nursing skills but increasingly uncomfortable with the unsafe environment in which I worked. We didn't have time to care for the eight to nine patients assigned to each of us. We didn't have enough support staff, management, or other necessary resources. Then came re-engineering, downsizing, and even larger patient loads, and my faith in the system faltered. With the assistance of the Illinois Nurses Association, several of us attempted to organize the nurses at our hospital. It was labor intensive and discouraging. During this period I also volunteered at the Champaign County Health Care Consumers (CCHCC), an award-winning grassroots organization working to improve local health care.

At one meeting, we were discussing the fact that both of the local hospitals claimed they were not for profit. Being fairly naive as to what that actually meant, the group explained the responsibilities that these hospitals had toward the community as a result of their tax-free status. They must provide a predetermined amount of charity work and community services. As the discussion went on, I thought about the situation at the hospital where I was working, and I was confused. I asked, "How can a hospital be not for profit when they outsource so many of their services to 'for profit' contractors?"

When asked to explain, I replied that my employer had hired contractors for the pharmacy, the dialysis unit, the rehabilitation department, the emergency room, dietary, and maybe more. There was silence in the room. The CCHCC director questioned me further and asked me to look into the matter and report back to the committee. Consequently, I started investigating by calling or visiting these various entities in the hospital and also their off-campus offices, such as the new medical building that would provide doctor's offices. Each and every one was for profit. The ER was staffed by a group of doctors out of Chicago who had formed a business of MDs for hire. The dialysis unit, even though on hospital property and staffed by our nurses, was owned and operated by the large, for-profit, dialysis company with headquarters on the east coast. Both the pharmacy and dietary also were owned and operated by outside agencies.

It appeared to those of us working with the CCHCC that a large percentage of the hospital was actually "for profit." Soon after I reported this to the committee, I took a traveling position at University of California, San Francisco, and CCHCC continued to investigate this problem and finally contacted the local tax authorities. CCHCC kept updating me about the ongoing investigation, and the Illinois Department of Revenue became involved. In 2003 the Illinois Department of Revenue ruled that the hospital was not providing enough charity care and would lose its tax-exempt status. Of course the hospital appealed, and the battles went back and forth. Illinois became the focus of this controversy, and nonprofit hospitals across the nation started being challenged.

In October 2008, the State Supreme Court refused to undo the Illinois Department of Revenue's decision to remove the hospitals tax-exempt status. This decision could cause the hospital to pay $6 million in back taxes. I have no idea if the hospital administration knows who started the investigation, but that does not really matter. What matters most to me is that my faith in human nature, in health care's duty to do what is right and honest and best for the patients and community was sorely damaged. I felt vindicated. They must have known what they were doing: turning away charity patients, outsourcing jobs outside the community, and illegally avoiding paying taxes that would have benefited the health care system of the town. I realized that one person, standing up for what is right, can sometimes make a difference.

So I continue working as a nurse, working with the California Nurses Association to improve patient care in California and beyond, fighting for universal health care through a bill for single-payer health care in my state, and most important of all, providing the best care for my patients and their families that is humanly possible in spite of the unsupportive environment in which we work.

· · ·

FAITH HENSON, RN, has worked as an RN, union organizer, and primarily a patient and nurse advocate in Illinois and California. In San Francisco she was an active CNA member and Chief Nurse Representative at a major San Francisco Hospital. She currently works as a hospice nurse in the Bay area.

A Safe Delivery from Domestic Abuse

Kristin Stevens

As a nurse midwife, I do more than deliver babies. I provide women's health care from menstruation through menopause; I follow women during pregnancy, helping them to prepare for the healthiest baby and best birth experience possible; and I follow women after they give birth to help them in their efforts to be healthy and prepared to meet the needs of their children. That's how I got to know Elena. She was in her early thirties, had two young children, and had recently delivered another. I had attended her during her last birth, and when she came to the hospital with her sick infant several months later, I was on duty when her baby was admitted to its pediatric unit.

The nurses on the floor alerted me that she and her baby were in the hospital, and I came over to check up on them. Over the course of a couple of days, I learned that Elena wasn't eating, was losing weight, and seemed depressed. I brought her food and talked with her over the next few days.

In our closing conversation, just before her baby was discharged, she said that she was distressed at home and worried about the other kids being at home with her husband. She didn't directly say there was any abuse, but even though she wouldn't tell me what it was, it felt to me like something was very wrong. We talked about abuse and I described what is okay and what isn't. I gave her information about the domestic violence hotline and told her people would help her if she ever felt she and her children were in danger of physical or verbal abuse. At that point I wasn't even thinking about sexual abuse. I tried to give her a lot of room to say what she needed to say, but she was still vague about what was happening. I knew she was under enormous stress and didn't have much family support or many friends whom she could rely on.

Two months later, Elena showed up in my office waiting room. Her baby and another of her children were with her. She was very distressed and confessed to me that not only was she at risk but she had also seen her husband engage in inappropriate sexual behavior with one of the children. We talked about that and agreed that she needed to leave the house and take her children with her. I knew that the best time for her to act was now, and so I suggested that perhaps she should leave today. She agreed. She arranged for someone to pick up her older child at school, and we talked about where she could stay. She could hardly speak—the effort to act without knowing what was going to happen was immense. She had not come into my office expecting not to return home that night.

I explained that she needed to call a hotline number to report the abuse and sat next to her while she did so. We were both glad I was there because as soon as she called the hotline, she was put on the defensive. Instead of listening to her explain her situation, the hotline staff interrogated her. "Why was she calling now? Why hadn't she called earlier? Why had she waited so long?"

She felt that she had to explain herself, as if she were somehow at fault rather than a victim. So not only did she talk to the people on the hotline, I also talked to them. I later notified the supervisor about how alarming it was to witness how she had been treated when she was doing the right thing in reporting the situation while she was personally in crisis.

We arranged a place for her to stay that night, and we called a women's shelter and arranged for her to go there with her family the next day. That night, I took her to the store to get what she needed overnight and then met her the next day at the shelter where she and her children would stay.

People there were very helpful. And, indeed, she ended up getting away from her husband and even went back to school, earning a nursing degree. She is now practicing as an RN.

I took a risk that afternoon suggesting that she and her children leave her home immediately. I knew if she went back home, with her meager support system, she might stay, and the abuse would only get worse. But I also knew that she had taken a risk in coming in and telling me her story. It was a risk that proved to be worth taking for us both.

. . .

Kristin Stevens, CNM, Ob-Gyn NP, has been involved in women's health care for more than thirty years. She currently provides GYN care for women in a primary-care practice in Ithaca, NY.

To Do the Unthinkable

Barry L. Adams

By 1996, the year *my* "trouble" started, the myriad reports that confirmed the extent of medical errors occurring in U.S. hospitals that were killing and injuring unsuspecting patients had yet to be written. The public, myself included, was not aware that there was, yet again, a looming shortage of registered nurses and the potential threat it posed to their health and safety. The nascent body of research that would eventually demonstrate consistently that RNs are critical to positive patient outcomes, including survival, could not yet be referred to as a "preponderance of scientific evidence." However, four years of actually practicing as an RN confirmed for me that indeed something was, in no small way, drastically wrong. That led me to do the unthinkable. I spoke up.

Why? I'm still not entirely sure. At age forty, I had never achieved anything that would deserve the label of "activist" or, most assuredly, "radical." As a gay man, who had survived the early years of the AIDS epidemic, I had, however, painfully learned that "silence equals death." I had also earned a credential and a professional license asserting that I was clinically competent and requiring me to protect the public. I was expected to do just that. So I did.

I was working at Youville Health Care Center, a rehabilitation hospital in Cambridge, Massachusetts, when I began to witness alarming problems with patient care. Suddenly, within only a couple of months, my own workload went from six to twelve patients. Other nurses were often caring for as many as sixteen patients. Under these conditions, we couldn't provide even basic nursing care. In one instance, I found a ninety-two-year-old stroke patient soaking in her own urine unable to reach the call button for help. Newly graduated nurses were left unsupervised to do complicated procedures, and potentially dangerous medication errors were increasing.

In accordance with both hospital policy and professional ethics, I tried to go through the proper channels and alert my superiors and engage my colleagues. That patients were in danger, and actually experiencing harm, was apparent to nearly every practicing nurse in every practice setting around the country. However, fear, uncertainty, and the prospect of hunger and no health insurance have a significant negative effect on discourse. Initially, I was ignored and later, blatantly threatened by nursing administrators. So I continued to do what I had always done, try to reduce risk to my patients and provide the best patient care I could. However, out of concern, I began reading the laws and regulations that governed nursing practice in Massachusetts. I looked more closely at what the state expected of health care institutions. I paid closer attention to the errors that were impacting patients on the unit, and I tried to identify patterns or practices that offered insight on how we could better reduce patient risk, particularly in the face of increasing patient care loads.

Again I attempted to work with the hospital's nursing administration, but with a more informed voice. However, after having received excellent personnel performance reviews that identified me as a "role model" for nursing, I suddenly was accused of having "time management problems" and behaving "unprofessionally." Ultimately, I was fired and then escorted out of the hospital by a security guard. Two other nurses who also spoke up about the deteriorating patient care were "disciplined." After facing similar allegations, they were suddenly mandated to work rotating night, day, and evening shifts, inflicting havoc on their personal and family responsibilities and school schedules.

Had we been part of a union, it is unlikely we could have been so arbitrarily disciplined. Even today I am disturbed by knowing that a collective bargaining contract may have protected our professional concerns for patient safety and possibly even prevented at least one accidental patient death that occurred the month I was fired. However, despite not having union protection, we chose to fight our case in "concerted effort" through the National Labor Relations Board (NLRB).

In 1997, after a two-day trial in Boston, a federal administrative law judge ruled that my termination was retaliatory and motivated by malice. He found that the evidence demonstrated that the hospital acted "to silence" us for disagreeing with the nurse administrators. Yet, only due to the willingness of the two nurses who were also retaliated against for speaking up were we able to make our point in a courtroom, not only once, but twice. The hospital appealed and lost a second time when the NLRB itself upheld the judge's initial conclusions. The result of three nonunionized nurses winning a well-documented case of retaliation before the NLRB was precedent setting. The publicity surrounding our case was significant, due to the efforts of both the Massachusetts Nurses Association (MNA) and the American Nurses Association, and continued from 1997 to 2000. Ultimately, the case was instrumental to successful passage of MNA's whistleblower legislation that protects all licensed health care providers in Massachusetts who report legitimate concerns for the safety of their patients.

What I have learned through all of this is that nursing requires intelligence, commitment, and a vision that allows one to see its essential human and social value. And that it's worth fighting for.

• • •

BARRY L. ADAMS, RN, is currently earning his doctoral degree at Brandeis University.

The Only Nurse
for Miles Around

Dagbjört Bjarnadóttir

I became a nurse in 1982 and spent my first years working in psychiatric wards, "regular" wards, and operating rooms. Eight years after my graduation, I was hired as a nurse at a health care clinic in central Iceland near Lake Mývatn, which is known for its exceptional natural beauty. The rural village I worked in had five hundred residents, who were mostly farmers. When I took the job, I was recently divorced and was alone with my school-age son. When I moved here, where I still work, I was the only health professional in the area. The health care center is a branch of a larger facility located in Húsavík, sixty kilometers (just under 40 miles) away. In Húsavík there are doctors and other nurses. Once a week, a doctor from Húsavík came to the clinic for consultations; otherwise, I was entirely—and still am—on my own. I found it exciting to experience situations that I hadn't encountered before and to face challenges in situations where my knowledge and resourcefulness would truly be tested.

I found that the workload was, and still is, very different in summer and winter. Lake Mývatn and its surroundings are known worldwide as a nature paradise, and it has become one of the most popular tourist attractions in Iceland. The influx of tourists into the surrounding wilderness during summer results in a wide range of problems from mosquito bites to serious accidents.

In contrast, winters by Lake Mývatn are tranquil, and there are hardly any tourists. But the weather can be ferocious, the roads inaccessible, and even impassable. My first years there, there were no mobile telephones, making communication more difficult. I have often been the first health care professional at the scene of an accident or serious illness. Under these conditions, it is imperative to read the situation correctly and make the right decisions quickly.

That's what I had to do at the end of a difficult day in the beginning of March 2001. I had decided to call my nurse supervisor in

Húsavík, whom I regularly call to get feedback about how I have solved problems. Because of my isolation, it is helpful to be in contact with other nurses. We were just about to hang up when I received a signal that someone was trying to reach the health clinic. Even though I was not on duty, I decided to answer the phone.

On the other end of the line was a very anxious father of a sixteen-month-old toddler. Of course I knew the family well, just as I know everyone near Mývatn. I had often visited them to follow up on the boy's growth, and the family came to the clinic for checkups and other problems. I had developed an emotional closeness to families that should never be underestimated, not only because it is therapeutically important but because it can be an extra burden for one nurse to carry.

The father said the child had been ill for a few days. He had a cold, a fever, and was lethargic. Shortly before he called me, he said, the boy had thrown up and now his situation had worsened; he seemed more ill and was unlike himself.

Under normal circumstances, I would have instructed the father to drive to the doctor on duty, all the way to Húsavík. My assessment of the situation was that the child needed assistance, now, not later! It was snowing, below freezing, with ice on the roads. It would have been too risky to send the child on a journey on the dark roads under these conditions without knowing what was wrong with him. So I went out to visit my young patient.

I was shocked when I saw him. He was pale and stiff, with the nape of his neck tilted slightly back. He was getting cramps that soon became very severe. His parents and sister were extremely anxious. Even though I too was nervous about misreading signs and symptoms, I took control of the situation right away. I gave the child medicine for the cramps and for the fever. I ordered the father to go to the clinic to get oxygen and told the mother to call for an ambulance right away to request that a doctor be sent with the ambulance. I called a children's specialist at the nearest pediatric ward, which is one hundred kilometers (about sixty miles) away in Akureyri. She agreed with everything that I had done.

The child's cramps lessened, but did not stop. I anticipated a difficult wait, since the ambulance could take up to an hour in this weather. The only thing for me to do during such a delay was to remain calm even though I was really scared to death. I worried about what would happen if the boy had another, more severe, cramp attack. What if the phone connection with the doctor was severed? Was I correct in remembering that the maximum dosage of cramp medicine for a child this age is x? How were the parents and sister going to react under this pressure? Would I be able to cope? In a small community like Mývatn, mistakes made during a crisis could destroy all the trust I had built up over the years.

We soon learned that an ambulance with a doctor was on its way from Húsavík. Shortly afterward another ambulance left the hospital in Akureyri with a pediatrician on board. The ambulance from Húsavík was closer. We were informed that the ambulance from Húsavík would drive us toward the ambulance from Akureyri, so that we could meet midway and get the child into the hands of a pediatrician as quickly as possible.

The child's vital signs were steady, and we gave him oxygen to help his breathing. Nevertheless I was worried because the cramping did not stop. An extra dose of the cramp medicine only helped temporarily, and the child was stiff, with his head tilted back. He rarely answered when spoken to. The pediatrician was very surprised by this and as we consulted over the telephone, we decided to give him an injection of the antibiotic Rocephin.

I found it difficult to inject a large dose of antibiotics in that small thigh, since he could react with discomfort and swelling to a dose that was too high. I therefore decided to divide the dose in two and injected half in each thigh. The boy showed almost no reaction to the injections. Finally, in just under an hour, the ambulance arrived.

With the boy, myself, and his mother on board, the ambulance sped off. Although she was nervous, the mother remained calm. The journey went well, oxygen saturation and vital signs were stable, but the boy still had cramps. After half an hour, we met the other ambulance, which took the boy and drove him to the children's ward.

I went home, and the next day the pediatrician from the hospital told me that the boy had improved and would recover, which was a great relief for me since I continued to worry about him throughout the night and early morning hours. He is now a healthy nine-year-old.

The people of Mývatn have come to trust me and, over the years, have thanked me for my work. My neighbors have demonstrated their trust and given me even more responsibility by electing me as a member of the city council. That's in addition to being their nurse.

· · ·

DAGBJÖRT BJARNADÓTTIR has worked in various health care institutions in Iceland (including surgical, pediatric, and psychiatric) and for the last twenty years has worked in the Lake Mývatn area in northern Iceland.

More Than Boo-boos and Band-Aids

Judy Stewart

When, after years as a pediatric critical care nurse, I became a school nurse in western Nebraska, I set out to transform the perception of the school nurse from one who puts Band-Aids on boo boos to one who plays a vital role in improving children's learning through health. I began with the idea that the school was my professional practice setting, all of the students and faculty were my client base, and the students, faculty, and families had the potential to be my "captive audience" during their public education experience. I also wanted to deal more assertively with the health issues students brought—increasing diabetes, obesity, the need to learn about sexuality—all these and more became part of my attempts to create a healthy student community.

My years of experience in the pediatric hospital setting quickly became the foundation for my care for students with chronic illness. Unfortunately, as the years passed, the incidence of chronic illness increased, and the current trends and research indicate the rates will rise to uncontrollable levels in the future. I manage my students' diabetic care, monitor blood sugars, manage hypo- and hyperglycemic events at school, teach families and students about diabetes, supporting them in learning to live with a chronic illness while being successful at school.

Diabetes is the tip of the proverbial iceberg. Among other things, I monitor, evaluate, and care for children with asthma, autism, attention deficit hyperactivity disorder (ADHD), muscular dystrophy, and cystic fibrosis. I developed my own system for early identification of mental health concerns with subsequent education, referral, and follow-up. I designed and implemented a school-based disease management program for my students—long before managed care demanded it. I have done all this by asking: Who are the champions that believe in health promotion who will transform our school into a healthy environment? The answer was crystal clear: the students! By mobilizing students, we were able, for example, to get rid of sodas in our vending machines.

My favorite program started after Christmas break. Realizing that I needed to lose twenty pounds to model healthy behavior for my students, I devised a staff weight loss program. My superintendent had problems with his knees, and I realized that he must lose seventy-five pounds before he could consider knee replacement. I gathered up my courage, collected my thoughts, reviewed my strategic plan, and entered into the superintendent's office. Sitting at his desk, this big burley man acknowledged my presence. I took a deep breath and asked, "Are you in a good mood?" "Why?" he growled. "Everyone in our hallway needs to lose weight, including me. We are going on a diet and exercise program. We will weigh in on Fridays. You gain—you pay money! See you Friday." I turned with relief and left his office.

On Friday, four of the five staff members showed up; we weighed and recorded our weights. Surprisingly, my superintendent arrived at my office and stepped on the scale. "You're right. I need to lose seventy-five pounds if I am going to have these knees replaced." WOW! The weeks passed, and we had our ups and downs, but in the end we were victorious. We all lost weight, and our superintendent lost the seventy-five pounds he needed to. He became a huge advocate of a healthy school environment, which fueled the process.

The healthy school environment idea caught on, and soon many people were calling and e-mailing the small school in western Nebraska for guidance and advice in creating their own healthy school environment.

Realizing how easy it was to stop vending soda, I decided to enter into the health policymaking arena. As a member of the Governor's Council for Health Promotion and Physical Activity, I addressed the possibility that Nebraska mandate that all schools vend only healthy beverages. What followed was a lesson in politics. After introducing the mandate, the following conversation ensued:

"Judy, what do we grow in Nebraska?"

Corn.

"What is the main ingredient in soda?"

High fructose corn syrup.

"Do you think Nebraska farmers will support this mandate?"

I remember thinking, why would corn production take precedence over the health of Nebraska's children? It makes no sense. In an instant I replied:

"Tell them to produce ethanol."

I learned that corn producers and soda companies are big strong bullies that entice schools into exclusive vending contracts. State Senator Arnie Stuthman introduced LB 285 prohibiting the sale of soda in schools. The bill never came out of committee. How could something so sensible be so difficult? Senator Stuthman persisted and was successful in passing a legislative resolution to study the problem of the sale of nonnutritious foods and beverages in schools. The resolution did progress to public hearing, with interesting results. There were a few people to speak in favor of the resolution, including Coke. Nebraska is a Pepsi state, so it was in Coke's best interest to stop the sale of soda in Nebraska schools. That's politics! The bill did not advance in Nebraska, but the soda companies soon came to the table in favor of vending bottled water and 100 percent fruit juice in schools.

Congress also passed PL 108.265 that requires all schools that participate in the free and reduced school lunch program to have a school wellness policy. This legislation places the responsibility for developing a wellness policy at the local level so that the individual needs of each district can be addressed. Unfortunately, there is no oversight or accountability. School nurses must continue to work within their school community to create public policy that creates a healthy school environment.

School nurses across America could all write a story like mine. But sadly, there are not many nurses in the schools across the United States. Healthy People 2010 recommends one school nurse for every seven hundred fifty students in every U.S. school, but the few of us that exist are spread very thin, often responsible for thousands of children. My colleagues and I are still fighting the image of boo-boos and Band-Aids so that policymakers, boards of education, and administration will realize the importance of the role of the school nurse in maintaining the health of children in America and preventing costly chronic health concerns with maintenance of quality of life.

• • •

JUDY STEWART, BSN, RN, BC, has been a school nurse in rural western Nebraska for twenty-five years and is Chair of the Governor's Council for Health Promotion and Physical Activity and past president of the Nebraska Association of School Nurses.

First Responders in the AIDS Epidemic

Richard S. Ferri

I do remember her office was hot, and wondering what the hell I was about to get myself into. It was before the days of mandatory air conditioning in hospitals and political correctness outside of them. Sweat was pouring down my back since I was obeying the new and insane rule that demanded nurse educators wear their lab coats at all times. I suppose the lab coat was the hospital's way of getting back at us for ditching the damn nursing cap.

It was 1984, and I was melting away in the outer office of the associate director of nursing at St. Vincent's Hospital in Manhattan. St. Vincent's Hospital School of Nursing had developed a worldwide reputation as being one of the finest diploma nursing programs in the world. Everyone knew that. Especially St. Vincent's grads. However, my suggestion that nursing caps were not necessary made me a newly minted "bad guy."

Everything was done at St. Vincent's because that was the way it was done . . . period. No need for discussion. I guess I nearly fatally wounded this sacred cow when, six months earlier, I very publicly supported a dress code change that did not *require* nurses to wear caps. I actually said I thought it was more important what a nurse put *in* her head rather than *on* it. I had blasphemed.

Aside from the heat, I was nervous as hell. I was about to shout off my mouth about a new disease that was killing gay men in our hospital. At first, this disease was called gay-related immunodeficiency disease (GRID), and now it was acquired immunodeficiency syndrome (AIDS). No matter what the name, I knew men were dying and no one was really noticing.

After a period of silent punishment, the director's secretary finally nodded, indicating I could enter the inner sanctum. As she pointed in the direction of the door, all I could think about was the munchkin screaming: "No one gets in to see the Wizard. No way! No how!"

However, the red-faced munchkin changed his mind when he heard Dorothy's story and announced: "Well, that is a horse of a different color!" I guess I was now a horse of a different color, but I felt more like a jackass.

The office was long, narrow, and windowless. Her desk was slammed against the wall, forcing her back to all who entered. She did not turn around, and I did not speak.

The puddles of sweat were now cascading down my back. She was the big-time nurse executive, and I was just the staff education instructor for critical care. We were not on a level playing field. Our paths had crossed rarely and usually harshly about the poor staffing of the intensive care unit. It hit me that I was just about to try to jump a fence, and I hadn't a clue in the world how to do it.

Somehow I found a slight voice and muttered, "I am here about all the AIDS in the hospital . . ."

I could see her shoulders fly up into an angry exclamation point as she said, enunciating every word, "I told you before we are not allocating any more aides to your unit!"

My mind did the quick mental gymnastics of decoding her intent and I cleared my throat again.

"I am talking about the new disease that is killing gay men right and left, not staffing."

She stopped and slowly turned around. She looked confused and unhappy. "What the *hell* are you talking about?"

"Sit," she pointed to a chair.

I sat.

"Talk," she commanded.

I talked for nearly half an hour, and she seemed to listen. I told her gay men, and now others, including heterosexual people, were contracting this newly discovered and ultimately fatal virus. People were becoming critically ill overnight and dying. No one had any real clue as to what the hell was going on.

After I said what I came to say, she just looked at me and said, "You are kidding me, right?"

"Sadly, no, I am not."

Her face turned scarlet once again, and she stood. "Take me for a walk around the hospital."

We left her office, and I walked her into the ICU and the ER to show her the half dozen or so young men in "prime health" hooked up to respirators and dying. All the men were in great physical shape, intubated, alone, and writhing in pain. The director touched each guy on the forehead as she rounded and asked the nurses to get them more morphine. I said nothing.

We walked out onto Seventh Avenue and stood in the sun. She looked up at me, and I could see her face begin to crumble.

Softly she said, "Thank you." And after a very long pause. "I had no idea."

I tried to shield my eyes from the sun, but frustrated tears started to form anyway. "That is the problem. No one does. No one has any idea we are in the middle of a gay Mecca and gay men are dying." Now I paused. "And dying scared, alone, and painfully."

She took my elbow and pointed me toward the Elephant and Castle café. After we were seated and ordered some wine, she leaned forward and said, "Here is the deal. You are to put together a mandatory in-service on this AIDS thing immediately. Get some local 'experts' and yourself to speak. Keep it to thirty minutes, and I will make sure every nurse, doctor, dietitian, and every other clinician attends." She finished off her glass of wine. I did the same.

"You let me know when you are ready and we will start to turn this mess around."

As we stood up to leave the café, I said, "I will be ready in two weeks or less. I have already been talking to people."

She almost smiled.

She went back to her office, and I went to mine—an old, dirty utility room tiled from floor to ceiling. I shut my office door and dunked my head under a sink of cold running water. I turned on the one little miserable fan I had and sat down and started to make my calls.

Eight days later, we held the first in-service with some local "experts" and the newly appointed "AIDS" liaison from the mayor's office. It worked. We ran the in-service around the clock to standing-room-only crowds.

An entire hospital community woke up to find themselves the first responders to the AIDS epidemic. Very few shied away. The majority of those nurses and doctors became unsung heroes in the middle of a brewing hell of one of the worst epidemics in history.

All it took was two nurses on opposite sides of the fence talking.

I never did think fences did any good. I still don't.

· · ·

RICHARD S. FERRI, PhD, ANP, ACRN, FAAN, practices HIV medicine on Cape Cod, and is the author of numerous text books, and peer-reviewed articles, in addition to being a published fiction writer and produced playwright.

Part 6

CHOKING ON SUGAR AND SPICE
Challenging Nurses'
Public Image

Almost every RN I've ever met has been concerned about the public image of nursing. Whether they're a nurse academic, a top-level administrator, a bedside RN, or an advanced practice nurse, most feel that non-nurses don't really understand what they do. When I give workshops or lectures, I always ask the audience two questions: (1) "How many of you think the public trusts nurses?" I could be in Chicago or Copenhagen, Toronto or Sydney, but every time, almost every hand in the room goes up. Then I ask the follow-up question: "How many of you think the public understands what nurses do?"

Invariably, no hands are raised. That's the paradox. The public trusts nurses but doesn't get what they do. People believe that doctors "know their stuff" (even when they don't), which is why, even though doctors score low on public trust surveys, people compliment them on their smarts. People similarly believe that nurses are sweet and nice (even though some of them aren't). What they don't know is that nursing is brain work not just heart work and that when nurses are at work, it's their minds not their emotions that are engaged.

Unfortunately, not enough nurses take advantage of the opportunities that present themselves, every day, to alter public misconceptions about nursing. In the sugar and spice narrative of nursing, showing how smart you are is definitely a no-no.

Consider the following example: An expert oncology nurse whose husband was a high-powered financial wizard (until the 2008 crash, that is) was attending a dinner party with her spouse. The guests and hosts were highly paid professionals and their spouses. One of these women turned to my friend over dinner and, dripping with conde-scension, said, "So I understand you're a nurse. Do you do it just to do a spot of caring?"

"What did you say to that?" I asked her.

"Nothing," she said.

Among friends, neighbors, or relatives, RNs may hear silly, inaccu-rate, or unflattering remarks about their profession. I can understand how frustrating and even disarming these encounters can be. While certainly not welcome, however, like the incident above, these are—if used correctly—"teachable moments."

In this section, several nurses show how they skillfully used such opportunities to confront common stereotypes about nursing—head on. What's especially significant about these stories is that the nurses who recount them didn't just stick up for their own slot or profes-sional silo. They claimed credit for what nurses do and spoke up for nursing in many different settings. Like Nurse Kozub, they spoke up for nurses in different fields, or, like Nurses Fagin, Shalof, or Grins-pun, for all nurses everywhere. They thus show that anyone—a nurse who heads an Ivy League university, a leader of a nursing organiza-tion, a bedside nurse chatting with friends—can help educate the public about what it needs to know about nursing.

Silenced during the SARS Epidemic

Doris Grinspun

Lights, camera, action!

Twelve nurses sat in two rows facing the journalists and politicians who had crowded into the Ontario government's media studio at Queen's Park in Toronto, Canada. When they were introduced by Adeline Falk-Rafael, the president of the Registered Nurses' Association of Ontario (RNAO), each nurse put on a surgical mask that had the word *ignored*, *silenced*, or *muzzled* written across it in black magic marker. For the next few minutes, the only sound in the room was the frantic clicking of camera shutters.

After months of having their voices ignored and discounted, nurses had found a dramatic way to deliver a powerful message to politicians.

It was June 2003, and an outbreak of severe acute respiratory syndrome (SARS) was entering its fourth month. This health crisis was unlike any other that the provincial government, health organizations, or health care professionals had faced before, and the impact was enormous. By June, the disease had claimed the lives of thirty-three people in Toronto, hospitalized hundreds of others, and quarantined tens of thousands. Tourism and travel to Toronto had dwindled, and the Ontario province was losing billions.

The SARS outbreak hit Toronto hospitals on March 7, 2003. A provincial emergency was declared on March 26 and lifted on May 18. Throughout this period, nurses were overworked and exhausted; stressful and unpredictable working conditions and fears of contracting the disease or infecting family members were taking a toll on their health and disrupting their personal lives. To make matters worse, the government had announced that the SARS outbreak was over—even with nurses' evidence and warnings to the contrary. Despite the government's announcement, anxious, frightened, and frustrated nurses began calling RNAO to report that they were still seeing new cases of the disease. Nurses at one hospital met with their manager to explain that people suffering from SARS were still coming into the emergency department. When the manager quickly arranged for the nurses to meet with the hospital's head of infection control, he humiliated and dismissed them by saying, "When I need an expert opinion, I ask the experts."

It turned out that the nurses were right. SARS wasn't over. In fact, the second wave of cases, which began on May 22—just four days after the provincial emergency was lifted—took the lives of two nurses and a physician. If health care organizations had heeded nurses' warnings, perhaps this second cluster of cases could have been prevented or at least diminished. Nurses were working in the eye of the SARS storm, but throughout the crisis their knowledge and expert opinions had been consistently disregarded and dismissed. No wonder they felt so angry, frustrated, and insulted.

To respond to nurses' concerns and the public health issues, we at the RNAO called the press conference to formally call on the government to order a full public inquiry into the outbreak of SARS. At the RNAO, we knew an inquiry of this type would be the only way to learn the following: how government, health care organizations, and health care professionals could have responded more effectively to the challenges of this outbreak; how we could better prepare for the next health care emergency; and why nurses' warnings were not heeded.

Two days after the press conference, the premier of Ontario announced an independent, full public review of SARS led by Justice Archie Campbell. It wasn't the full public inquiry we had called for, which would have included cross-examination, but it did include the whistleblower protection that RNAO had demanded and other important provisos. It was a victory for nurses and others who dared to speak truth to power.

Several lessons were learned from the SARS outbreak. I'm still deeply troubled by what the crisis taught me: that health care organizations did not recognize nurses as knowledge workers and, therefore, did not respect their views or advice or take them into consideration. Professional associations such as the RNAO encourage and support nurses to speak up about their clinical expertise so health care organizations and the public will understand that this expertise goes far beyond nurturing. During SARS, nurses followed this advice, but their voices were ignored, silenced, and muzzled.

Nurses couldn't help but wonder if the decision to lift the state of emergency was a political exercise to appease the business community rather than a public safety directive meant to protect the public and health care professionals. The World Health Organization (WHO) had issued a travel advisory for Toronto on April 23, and while it was rescinded on April 29, Toronto's SARS outbreak was still making news internationally, and many people were afraid to travel to the city. Even local residents were staying away from restaurants and other public places for fear of contracting the disease. SARS was not only a serious health concern; it was bad for business.

During the SARS crisis, nurses discovered that their clinical expertise did not guarantee that they would be listened to or taken seriously. Media savvy was required to communicate with politicians and other decision makers. We finally made our voices heard, but it shouldn't have taken so much effort. Society needs to fundamentally change the way they view and treat nurses (which is also the way they view and treat women) and the way nurses participate in the labor force. Nurses also have a key role to play in bringing about these systemic changes. At every opportunity, we must speak of the clinical, organizational, and system knowledge and skills we bring to our work, the difficult activities we engage in, and the procedures we perform. Collectively we can—and we must—create an authentic image of our extraordinary profession.

· · ·

DORIS GRINSPUN, RN, MSN, PhD (cand), O.ONT, is the Executive Director of the Registered Nurses' Association of Ontario, has received numerous professional and scholarly awards, and in 2003 was invested with the Order of Ontario, which recognizes the highest level of individual excellence and achievement in any field.

In the Halls of Academe

Claire M. Fagin

When you've been in nursing for as long as I have—over sixty years—the times you've had to stand up for the profession are too numerous to count. Recall the adage: If I only had a penny for every . . . Rather than collecting pennies, I've collected a lot of lessons. Over time, I have distilled them into three major themes: (1) Alliances are essential, including getting support from those outside the profession; (2) You should always put the needs of patients in the forefront; and (3) At times, you should be prepared to play hardball and not back down.

Although I have thousands of stories to choose from in my long career of standing up for nursing, here's one that illustrates these points.

In 1969, I was asked to start a baccalaureate nursing program at Lehman College, which is part of the City University of New York (CUNY). When I got there, the program had to get faculty approval, and I went to the faculty meeting where that was discussed. As I sat there, the chairman of the Sociology Department stood up to speak. "Why on earth would we want to approve a nursing program here?" he asked. "Nurses are only maids. They empty bedpans. We don't need a program like that at this school. Why would we want such a low-class program?"

I was shocked. I knew the college and the president wanted the program. I gathered myself together and stood up. "Let me ask you something professor," I said, "Have you ever been a patient in a hospital?"

"No," he said.

"Well," I continued, "I hope you aren't anytime soon because if that's what you think you're going to get from nursing, you're not going to get well in that hospital."

When I sat down, the head of the program that supported the educational advancement for minority students stood up and read the sociology chairman the riot act. Our program was approved, and he later became, if not a pal, at least a supporter.

But that wasn't the only hurdle we had to confront. About two years later, after I had recruited excellent faculty and launched the program, but before we had graduated our first class, I heard via the grapevine that the surgeons at nearby Montefiore Hospital wanted Lehman College to start a degree-granting physician assistant (PA) program to train PAs to take over nurses' work in the operating room and to substitute for medical residents on the floors.

Our students in the first baccalaureate program to include such skills were being educated as primary care practitioners. Although we were becoming well recognized, we had not yet tested our model, and I found the notion of preparing PAs at Lehman unacceptable. I told the vice provost for academic affairs about my concerns, and she promised her support.

Because the doctors knew of my opposition to their program, the chief operating officer (COO) of the hospital called to invite me to lunch. Naturally, I accepted. I went to meet him at a well-known Italian restaurant. As I walked up, black stretch limos were disgorging celebrity diners. The place was extraordinary, and we had a superb meal. And then, of course, the COO got to the point and told me essentially to back off. And I said I wouldn't do it.

"Look," I told him, "the lunch was delicious and wonderful. But you can't wine and dine me to get me to support this program. You can't buy me with lunch, or with anything else," I added.

He had failed, so now the surgeons tried. They invited me to a meeting and, knowing I had the support of the vice provost and the president, I told them that they should not go ahead with their program and at least wait a couple of years until our first class had graduated. I made it clear that I would not support their bid to create a PA program within Lehman College. And then I made a deal with them.

I said that our graduates were going to be prepared to do the kind of work they wanted. My program was preparing nurses for primary care practice, and it was the first in the country to do that. I told them that my med-surg faculty would spend the summer at Montefiore acting as residents and that after this one summer they would take the PA exam. So they agreed, and then I had to convince the faculty to do the same. Which I did. So several Lehman nursing faculty, including Ellen Baer and Shirley Stokes Green, spent the summer working as residents. And it went very well except that the PA association wouldn't let them take the exam.

Lehman did not approve the PA program, and it was later started at another college.

After I left Lehman College to become dean of the University of Pennsylvania School of Nursing, I faced many more dilemmas and challenges and was able to help and support advancements in nursing education and research that have benefited and will continue to benefit patients and nurses for years to come. In 1993, the chairman of the board of the university, Alvin Shoemaker, appointed me as interim president of the University of Pennsylvania, and I held that position for a year. I was the first nurse and woman in the United States to be the chief executive officer of an Ivy League university. After I left, two women—first Judith Rodin and then Amy Guttmann—followed as presidents of Penn. (Now there are many women presidents of universities, including four in the Ivy League.)

In 2008, I was invited to a celebration honoring Alvin Shoemaker, a true pioneer. After a moving program about his accomplishments, he commented on his Penn experience and the things that had been said about him that evening. With a twinkle in his eye, he said, "You know, when I appointed Claire Fagin as interim president, I was tickled to do so and have all those doctors reporting to a nurse."

So was I.

. . .

CLAIRE M. FAGIN, PhD, RN, is Dean Emerita, Professor Emerita, School of Nursing, Claire M. Fagin Hall, University of Pennsylvania.

R-E-S-P-E-C-T

Lisa Fitzpatrick

Every three years in the state of Victoria, the Australian Nursing Federation (ANF) (Victorian Branch [VB])—the union that represents approximately 49,000 nurses of whom 28,000 are employed in 110 Victorian State government–run health facilities (a mixture of hospitals, nursing homes, and community health centers)—has to negotiate a legally binding enterprise agreement that determines the entire terms and conditions of employment for the next three years. It also sets the agenda for other nurses and midwives employed in other sectors throughout Victoria. The agreement is negotiated with representatives of the health facilities and the Victorian State government. I'm the state secretary of our union and a nurse with twenty-nine years of experience.

In 2000, our union won the first nurse-to-patient ratios in the country. Winning those ratios was not easy. Maintaining them has also required constant action and vigilance.

To win ratios in 2000, nurses decided to close one in four of the beds in all medical and surgical wards in the Victorian health system. So, how exactly did the nurses "close the beds?" And why did management of the health facilities and the Victorian State government allow it?

Audaciously, once a patient is discharged, a "Bed Closed" sign is placed on the pillow by a nurse, and, on occasion, the mattress is hidden. Patients are not admitted to these beds by nursing staff. To ensure that genuine emergencies were able to be admitted into a nominally "closed bed," the nurses also closed an additional two beds on each ward that were able to be opened if the circumstances genuinely warranted it. Extraordinarily, this was mostly carried out without hindrance from the hospital management. If a health facility attempted to force an admission into a "closed bed," nurses threatened to increase the numbers of beds that would be closed in that facility, and that was usually sufficient. Importantly, nurses remained at work, continued to be paid, and patients in hospital were well cared for. Further, the nurses proved that they could professionally assess a genuine emergency and flexibly apply the "closed bed" rules without jeopardizing patient safety. It would not be unreasonable to speculate that health facility management did not wish to challenge nurses on patient safety issues in circumstances where nurses would have a myriad of tales exposing administrative incompetence that had previously led to patient safety issues.

In 2004, the union had to wage a campaign to protect the ratios. This was my first EBA campaign in my capacity as the union state secretary. We utilized the "closed beds" strategy to great effect then and maintained the ratios. The ANF (VB) elected to further refine their strategies for the 2007 enterprise agreement, building on the successful foundations of the "closed beds" industrial campaign with a sophisticated media and new technologies campaign. In an early negotiation meeting with the state government, ANF (VB) officials saw a document that indicated the state government was planning to again attempt to abolish nurse-patient ratios, and that the media slogan for the state government campaign would be "Nursing—For a Better State of Health."

The ANF (VB) decided to ambush the limitless financial capacity of the state government by launching a campaign titled "Fund Nursing Properly—For a Better State of Health." It included all aspects of traditional media outlets such as newspapers, television, and radio, as well as the Internet and social networking sites such as MySpace and Facebook. The ANF (VB) leadership recognized that younger nurses were more likely to support the old style "bed closed" campaign with a blend of technological supports such as e-mail and mobile phone text messaging that were unheard of at the time of the original 1997 conception of the "bed closed" campaign.

In October 2007 nurses once again voted unanimously to take industrial action in support of better workloads, improved nurse/midwife-patient ratios, salaries, and working conditions. An important legislative change concerning the rights of Australian workers had recently been enacted in March 2006—the now ousted conservative federal governments' "WorkChoices" industrial legislation was in place. This time, despite nurses' remaining at work and performing their duties, the WorkChoices legislation demanded that employers dock the pay of those nurses participating in the bed closure action for a minimum of four hours each day or for the employers to be fined themselves.

Within three days, nurses had closed 1,300 beds throughout the state of Victoria. Public support of the nurses' action remained high, and the government representatives were forced to sit down at the negotiating table with the union and take the nurses' demands seriously. As expected, the nurses' action was deemed to be unlawful, and the government sought to prosecute the union and its officials in Australia's federal court. Despite this action, the nurses and their union stood united.

The union utilized an important forum to facilitate communication to and among nurses and supporters: the Internet. Thousands of messages were logged on the "fund nursing properly" website (www.fundnursingproperly.com), and the state government politicians were forced to answer tough media questions arising from the recording of nurses' daily experiences. Using the Internet, nurses in remote rural hospitals could share their experiences with nurses from major metropolitan hospitals. One key theme that emerged was that the dispute wasn't just about the money and workloads for the nurses—it also was about respect. Nurses certainly wanted improved employment conditions, but respect and recognition were just as important.

After nine days and nights, over five thousand nurses and midwives attended a meeting to consider the state government's offer that had been negotiated by the union. They marched into the meeting to the applause of hundreds of unionists from other unions and the voice of Billy Bragg singing "There is power in the union."

During the bed closure action, thousands of nurses had their pay docked, and the ANF (VB) started a welfare fund to which people could donate through the "fund nursing properly" website. One hundred and eighty thousand dollars was given out to nurses who found themselves in financial difficulty as a result of not receiving any pay for the nine days (even though the nurses had been at work the whole time!). But nurses and midwives believed it was all worth it.

The agreement provided wage increases of between 16 and 30 percent over four years and improved nurse-patient ratios in emergency departments and postnatal wards. Importantly, the nurse-patient ratios won in previous disputes were kept. An additional three hundred nurses would be employed to help relieve workload pressures in other areas. The agreement improved a number of other employment entitlements, such as paid maternity leave.

The nurses left the meeting singing along to Aretha's anthem—"R-E-S-P-E-C-T."

Two thousand five hundred nurses joined the ANF (VB) during the three-month campaign. Forty-eight percent of those nurses were under the age of thirty-five. A new generation of Victorian nurses had learned how to close beds and for the first time had experienced the power of collective action.

Here, for example, is a comment from a young nurse posted on the "fund nursing properly" website on October 25, 2007, the day the dispute was settled and Victorian nurses won some RESPECT. She says, "As a graduate, this was very new to me. . . . I have received so much support and education about everything. . . . WELL done to all the nurses who stood together, united, undefeated."

• • •

LISA FITZPATRICK, RN, a Registered Division 1 nurse from Melbourne, Australia, has been the State Secretary of the ANF (Victorian Branch) since 2001 and in 2009 was re-elected for a third term; in 2001 she was awarded the Australian Centenary medal for her outstanding contribution to the Victorian union movement.

Real Nurses Don't Wear Wings

Victoria L. Rich

Throughout my career, I have always been concerned with the issue of nursing image. How we, as nurses, appear to others, I am convinced, is a reflection about how we feel about ourselves and how we judge our own importance. Since bedside nurses abandoned the white cap and starched white uniforms, however, nurses' image in the workplace has gone from rigidly circumscribed to pretty much anything goes. When, before 2005, I walked around the hospital I'm privileged to lead, the Hospital of the University of Pennsylvania (HUP), I saw nurses in white coats, nurses in tailored, one-color scrubs, nurses in T-shirts with their belly buttons in full view, and nurses in scrub tops decorated with Snoopy, Smurfs, and angels. I knew that the people I saw in these outfits were nurses. But few others—particularly patients and physicians—shared that critical knowledge because many other categories of workers wore similar outfits. Unfortunately, I'd been unable to do much to change it until I was presented with the "perfect storm" of events in 2004.

Our hospital system as a whole was addressing the issue of creating a more respectful workplace. One of our major concerns was nurse/physician collaboration. Because of increasing volumes of patients in the hospital and a national nursing shortage, we found that people were experiencing a lot of stress and compassion fatigue, which seemed to be translating into a lack of collaboration and communication between doctors and nurses. Because our hospital was seeking Magnet accreditation—a program developed by the American Nurses Credentialing Center (a subsidiary of the American Nurses Association) to recognize hospitals that provide nursing excellence—we were looking at our quality indicators. The National Database for Nursing Quality Indicators (NDNQI) told us that one of our lowest scores was in the area of physician-nurse collaboration.

Because of this, I was able to go to the hospital executive team as well as to physician leadership in the hospital and discuss the issue with them. The dean of the medical school, Dr. Arthur Rubinstein, was also concerned about these issues, and the University of Pennsylvania Medical School had similarly set up a respectful workplace committee on which I sat. As we talked in this group, it became clear that no one knew with whom they were working on the floors. People didn't know who was a doctor, a nurse, a nurse's aid, a respiratory therapist. People rarely said, "Hello, I'm Doctor so and so, or I'm Nurse so and so." Name tags were almost always turned front to back. In fact, lots of people didn't even wear name tags. And uniforms were no longer identifiers of a professional or occupational group.

When I walked out of these committee and I looked at how the nurses were dressed, all I saw was a mishmash of anonymity. Well, I thought, I can't control the physicians in this organization, but we, as RNs, can control who we are and how we present ourselves.

From my studies of complexity theory, I knew about the so-called 15 percent rule: If you want to change a culture or organization, you don't focus on the whole 100 percent, on everything that needs change; you focus on the one or two things you think you can actually change. How we present ourselves at work, I believed, was one of these things. We needed to be easily identifiable as nurses and all wear the same uniform.

Putting that theory into action wasn't easy. Even though we, as nurses, often complain that we don't get enough respect, that patients don't know who we are, and that doctors don't ask us about our concerns, when I broached the idea of a uniform change to HUP nurses, they were quite resistant. They felt they had a right to express their individuality at work by wearing—within limits—whatever kind of uniform they wanted to wear. They felt that because they are independent professionals, no one should tell them what to wear.

How could I convince them that if we really believe that we are the most important person to the patient, we have to wear the garb that conveys our hard-earned professional stature? After all, we, like police and firefighters, are critical to patient safety and rescue. They are identifiable. Why aren't we?

We had many meetings on this subject at HUP. I discussed the issue with the nursing staff as well as at the nursing shared governance committee that included thirty-five leaders chosen by each unit in the hospital. We had experts in nursing image come and speak, and we conducted an online survey about the issue. We finally got nurses to agree that they should all wear one colored uniform. The nurses themselves decided on the color—navy blue. We also decided to embroider a symbol on these navy blue scrubs—the symbol for the HUP nursing model of excellence and professional practice. Because people still wanted to maintain a sense of individuality, nurses decided to not only put RN on the uniform but also identify the unit they worked on—for example, the cardiothoracic unit, neurosurgery, oncology.

After this consensus building came the issue of cost. "How much would this cost nurses who had already purchased a stock of uniforms?" I asked. Since nurses were also concerned about cost, I was determined that this important issue not get in the way of success in this effort. So I went to our CEO, who, along with many of the physicians, was committed to the idea that nurses should be easily identified. (Some of the physicians even suggested that we go back to whites with caps. "No way is that ever going to happen," I said, putting an end to that idea.)

To the CEO and COO, I proposed that we purchase every one of our 1,500 registered nurses two scrub uniforms. Whenever we hired a nurse, he or she would receive two uniforms as a welcome gift. In order to do this, however, we had to get our CEO and COO not only to agree to this financial outlay but to help us deal with other hospital departments. Many staff in other departments—such as surgical techs and instrument staff in the perioperative area—wore navy blue scrubs. If nurses were to be identified by their navy blue, then respiratory and surgical technicians or transport workers couldn't wear them as well. The CEO and COO agreed. They would do what it took to ensure that only RNs at HUP would wear navy blue. Their willingness to make such an agreement allowed me to go back to our nurses with a powerful message: Look how much this organization is prepared to invest to underscore the importance of nursing at HUP.

Over the next months, we worked with nurses to discuss what fabric the uniforms would be made of. We invited uniform manufacturers into the hospital to put on fashion shows so nurses themselves could decide which material and style of uniform they preferred. All RNs, including the nursing leadership team and myself, wear navy blue scrubs when rounding on the units. Nurse unit managers and leaders on the shared governance committee agreed to speak with nurses who didn't show up to work in navy blue.

After two years of work, RNs in our organization have really embraced this change. About ten times a year, I receive an e-mail from a HUP nurse telling me that she—or he—has had a family member admitted to another hospital. Invariably they tell me that it's impossible to figure out who is—and who is not—a nurse. "Victoria," they write, "when we started all this, I really didn't believe in it. But now, after my own experience elsewhere, I realize how important it is to be able to easily identify an RN." Not only has HUP changed; RNs at our sister institution, Presbyterian Hospital, and Pennsylvania Hospital all now wear navy blue. Moreover, RNs in the majority of our 125 ambulatory practices now wear navy blue. We have also gotten many letters from patients telling us how much they appreciate being able to easily identify nurses, and we've received positive comments from physicians.

Perhaps the most compelling evidence of how important this change has been occurred in fall 2008, when we had a fire on the twelfth and fourteenth floors at HUP. In the midst of the smoke, blaring alarms, and chaos, we had to safely evacuate seventy-five patients. The process went very smoothly. When we debriefed about what had happened, everyone identified a key factor that helped determine a successful outcome: Because all the nurses were in navy blue, critical players in this evacuation were easy to spot. In a true disaster, everyone ended up safe in large part because everyone knew who was a registered nurse.

· · ·

Victoria L. Rich, PhD, RN, FAAN, is Chief Nurse Executive, University of Pennsylvania Medical Center, Chief Nursing Officer, Hospital of the University of Pennsylvania, Associate Executive Director, Hospital of the University of Pennsylvania, Associate Professor, Nursing Administration, University of Pennsylvania School of Nursing.

The Lady with a Loud Voice

Jeanne Bryner

In the pantheon of nursing, "the lady with a lamp"—the fabled Florence Nightingale—looms large as a teller of tales about the lives and work of nurses more than a century ago. In the new millennium, the voices of rank-and-file RNs are often lost in mass media coverage that downplays or ignores the role of nondoctors in health care systems.

In 2004, I tried to remedy this problem by publishing *Tenderly Lift Me: Nurses Honored, Celebrated, and Remembered*. The book includes poems by me and first-person accounts by nurses that try to alleviate some of the prevailing ignorance and confusion about our profession's past, present, and future.

Unbeknownst to her, the late South Carolina nurse-midwife Maude Callen led me to this unusual project. When I had my first writing fellowship, I stumbled across Maude's story in the bound periodical section of a university research library. W. Eugene Smith had photographed this amazing woman who served her community in the rural South until the very day of her death. Inspired by Maude, I wrote a sonnet that is now a song as well. And when people ask me how I chose the nurses profiled in my book, I tell them, "They chose me." For example, I'd be recycling a newspaper and find a small photo of a nurse or a vignette about a senior citizen who also was a nurse. These items would catch my eye, and I'd begin to investigate further.

I approached my writing the way I approach my life: with curiosity. How did people come to be nurses? What do other people need to know about nurses? What made nurses choose to leave the field or continue in their profession? What external forces fracture our world to shape our lives? What did the face of nursing look like years ago and how does it appear now? I wanted a diverse cast of characters in my book, and I wanted to address the ongoing global problems and concerns of RNs, because our work has no domestic or international borders.

How could I possibly know, as a white woman from Appalachia, what it meant to be born black in rural Alabama in 1921, until I interviewed Helen Albert? Part of the great African American migration north, Helen was the first black registered nurse ever hired in Trumbull County, Ohio. From the poignant stories of her youth, I learned that southern segregation was not just a system of legal subjugation. It was a sordid and soiled regional laundry, in which human beings were routinely sorted into their respective piles: whites here, darks over there. Segregation was a label maker for separate but unequal drinking fountains, bathrooms, and schoolhouses. I listened to Helen as she relived her long, hot days spent working in cotton fields, while also assisting the family of her hometown's white physician—a connection that later facilitated her professional education as a nurse. Throughout our interviews, I was struck by Helen's matter-of-fact tone.

Because of her race, Helen was not accepted to nurse's training when she first applied. A year later, her former employer, Dr. Martin, spoke to school officials, and she was finally admitted. Helen ultimately graduated first in her class but failed the state boards on her first try, proving that one test score does not a life make, for she succeeded on her next try. An internationally recognized RN, Helen did not retire until she reached the age of eighty-seven, after sixty years of distinguished nursing and community service.

A nurse colleague introduced me to eighty-three-year-old Esther Gundry. Esther lived in a tidy little house less than thirty miles from me, where she was the loyal keeper of her Aunt Jenny's World War I nurse photo album, mess kit, engraved canteen, and forks. Esther was more than happy to share the story of her family's migration from Wales to a coal-mining community in Pennsylvania. She dug out family photos of Jenny and told me stories about the premature deaths of her parents. The orphaned child and her four sisters were all eventually adopted, but only Jenny received a formal education. With Aunt Jenny's photo album spread across our laps, afternoons slipped into evenings as Esther and I read Jenny's poignant handwritten comments in the margins: "He [a pilot] made the supreme sacrifice," "my best friend in the fracture ward," "Pershing here to visit." Jenny's careful notations were written for those who would come later. They were written for us. I'd drive home from Esther's house wondering about the fate of British soldiers lying in a field hospital, casualties of a foreign war, and about the young nurses who cared for them, as Nightingale had in an earlier European conflict.

A pure stroke of luck put a retired Irish-born nurse in the same emergency room where I worked. I always talk to my patients. If they are retired, I ask them about what jobs they did. When I asked Nora Mary Carmody McNicholas this question, she leaned over and said, "You'll not believe this, but I was a nurse." Her green eyes sparkled, and we became friends. I visited her in the hospital and later at the assisted living facility that became her final home. Nora had crossed the Atlantic to America, by herself, at the tender age of fourteen. She came to the profession later in life. It was only when her last child was a preteen that she decided to become a nurse. At age fifty, she began her studies and succeeded in getting a degree. Many of our conversations were about displacement. Nora still had her brogue and, to me, it was music. But, for her, it seemed to be a burden, an unwanted ethnic brand. Nora spoke proudly of her college-educated children and grandchildren, but when she spoke of her homeland, it was always with a tinge of sadness, weighed down by memories of the past. "Ireland is a beautiful country, but very poor. It's green there, but Father could never find enough work." Nora's voice would drift off, and she'd let out a deep sigh that filled the room. I believe it was a last expression of grief for her mother's fatal cough, her lost girlhood, and her now-forlorn village of abandoned fields, old thatched roof houses, and falling-down walls.

Nurses are human, too, and thus as fragile as the people we care for, although not while on the job. Through these stories, I want readers to know who we were and are, under the difficult conditions of health care work, past and present. We are not firefighters or police officers but, no less than these brave men (and yes, they are still mostly male), we rescue, protect, and serve. It was my privilege to hear and record the stories of brave nurses overcoming racial inequalities, physical disability, the burdens of family responsibilities, the dangers of war, and continuing discrimination against women.

• • •

JEANNE BRYNER, RN, CEN, has been a nurse for thirty years and is a graduate of Trumbull Memorial Hospital School of Nursing and Kent State University's Honors College.

Taking on the Terminator

Vicki Bermudez

In 2004, nurses in California started rallying, carrying signs against Governor Arnold Schwarzenegger when he tried to derail a bill guaranteeing patients safe nurse-to-patient ratios. Nurses in California were getting press coverage throughout the country. Some nurses felt that we might not look "proper" or "professional" in the eyes of the public. I was then working as the California Nurses Association (CNA) regulatory policy specialist. As I was having coffee with a nurse executive with whom I had worked during the legislative session, she asked me point blank whether what we were doing helped nursing's public image.

It was pretty clear that what CNA nurses were doing didn't fit with nursing's past image as physician's handmaidens subject to both physician and employer whims or to the medical model that is often held up as the benchmark of professionalism.

What nurses were doing was trying to protect the first licensed nurse-to-patient ratio legislation to be passed in the United States. After a ten-year struggle, the bill was passed and signed in 1999. But it wasn't until January 2004—following a study of California hospital staffing standards and the long California Department of Health Services (CDHS) administrative rule-making process—that the ratios were implemented. The first ratios were to begin in January 2004, with improved ratios phased in January 2005 and 2008.

Two months before implementation, all California administrative rule making was suddenly and unexpectedly suspended by the newly elected Governor Arnold Schwarzenegger, who had successfully replaced the recalled Governor Gray Davis, the governor who had signed the ratio bill into law. Since the ratio administrative process had been finalized September 26, 2003, prior to the election, the ratio regulations were allowed to go forward despite heavy political pressure from the hospital industry to scuttle the regulations as part of the governor's wholesale review of administrative agency functions. The ratio regulations managed to survive the first challenge in a new administration.

Only days before the January first implementation, the California Healthcare Association (CHA) filed a lawsuit against the CDHS alleging that a "Frequently Asked Questions" document that had been prepared by CDHS created a new and unexpected requirement that the minimum ratios had to be maintained even during meals and breaks. CNA joined the CDHS in its fight to defend the infant ratios against the hospitals' newest wrinkle in its years'-long attempts to undermine the law. The lawsuit ended after five months, on May 24, 2004, in a decision in which Superior Court Judge Gail Ohanesian stated, "applying the ratios to break periods is not new, and it is consistent with the plain language of the regulation. Any other interpretation would make the nurse-to-patient ratios meaningless."

The ratios regulations had withstood the second challenge, but we knew that the hospital industry would be undeterred. When, on November 4, we learned that "emergency regulations" had been filed that would prevent the 2005 phase-in of the medical-surgical ratios and undermine ratio enforcement in emergency departments, it still came as a shock. The court decision against CHA was only six months old, and the ratios themselves had not yet reached their first anniversary. The evidence the CDHS had of an "emergency" that required their intervention was newspaper evidence gathered in response to the press release campaign that CHA itself had devised. This final outrage drove CNA nurses into statewide protests and into the courts once again. This time, however, CNA was suing the agency it had recently partnered with in the lawsuit against the CHA. This was definitely a first.

The lawsuit, a writ of mandamus, was filed by CNA, and thousands of pages of evidence, declarations, and briefs were submitted to Superior Court Judge Judy Hersher. The governor, the CDHS, and the CHA attorneys worked together on the same side against the California Nurses Association. In my role as the regulatory policy specialist and RN, I prepared declarations for CNA's attorney that were submitted to the court explaining the California Nurse Practice Act, the role of the RN in providing safe patient care in the hospital

setting, and the significance of the nurse-patient relationship including nurses' obligation under law to act as a patient's advocate. The
ratio law regulatory process had thousands of pages of documents
that needed to be reviewed. Adobe Acrobat's "search" function became my new best friend; the state archives, my new office; and the
twelve-minute slow jog to the court from the CNA office, where volu-
minous documents were filed, a regular source of exercise.

The administrative agency (in this case the CDHS) is generally
given the benefit of the doubt when it comes to interpreting a statute,
and courts are reluctant to substitute their interpretation of a law
for that of the agency. This usually means that it is an uphill battle for
anyone suing an agency over its regulations. Fortunately, there are
also legal precedents that limit some of the actions of an agency-run-
amok and that make the court the final decision maker over the legal
interpretation of a statute.

In a carefully worded decision on CNA's petition for injunctive relief pending a final decision by the court, Judge Hersher granted the
injunction on March 4, 2005, stating that the CDHS had relied on
hearsay testimony obtained from newspaper articles and that the
agency admitted in its "Finding of Emergency" that it did not even
know if the reports were true. The court determined that the agency
had abused its authority and that the determination of "emergency"
was arbitrary, capricious, and lacking in evidentiary support. For
those reasons the court believed that there was a strong likelihood
that CNA would prevail in its claim in the final determination. In effect, the medical-surgical ratios of one RN to five or fewer patients
at all times would immediately go into effect in all hospitals (albeit
three months late), and all of the ER requirements returned to their
pre-emergency regulation status while a final determination was
made about the lawsuit or "writ." I read the decision and sat in court
stunned over the magnitude of the victory over the agency, the governor, and the hospital association. I knew the importance of this decision to patients and to the nurses who cared for them.

The final ruling, a brilliantly reasoned thirty-three-page decision
upholding CNA's petition to invalidate (enjoin) the emergency regulations came two months later after reams of legal arguments and
evidence had been submitted to the court.

I have read the decision too many times to count, but each time I read it, I thrill at the memory of nurses demonstrating against the injustice of a government willing to harm patients as a favor to hospital contributors and a governor who believed that his Hollywood popularity would insulate him from the wrath of the nurses whose hard-won victories for safe patient care had been snatched from them in political gamesmanship.

In my forty years as a registered nurse, I have always felt that the most satisfying professional experiences I have had have been at a patient's bedside. Although my part was small and I was involved mostly in the court action, the satisfaction I felt for the triumph of the California Nurses Association over administrative manipulation ranked up there with the most satisfying of all my professional life. Whoever said, "you can't beat city hall" didn't know about the power of nurses acting together. California has a governor who learned the hard way that it is not a safe political place to be when you stand between the nurses and their patients.

· · ·

VICKI BERMUDEZ, RN, a direct care nurse for over thirty years, was Labor Representative and Regulatory Policy Specialist for California Nurses Association and currently works in Neonatal Intensive Care at Kaiser Foundation Hospital in Roseville, California.

Defending the Nursing Profession over Dinner

Elizabeth Kozub

The table was lush with food: the caramelized carrots, candied yams, green bean casserole, and, of course, the fifteen-pound turkey, elegantly basted and cooked to perfection. We gathered around the table to celebrate Thanksgiving with some of our closest friends and coworkers, none of them nurses. The conversation flowed from one topic to another, eventually leading to gossip that a colleague, not present at the dinner, had a "natural childbirth." I asked, "Really, so there was nobody assisting in the childbirth?" One person at the table, often known for his boisterous opinions, exclaimed, "It was just a midwife, or something like that; there weren't even any doctors there."

I'm not a nurse midwife. I work in an intensive care unit. So I could have chosen to just let this comment slide by. But every time someone says something demeaning about one category of nurses, it hurts all nurses no matter where they work. I decided I couldn't just let his comment stand. Nursing needed to be made visible here, and I was the only who could do it.

Given that none of the other people was a nurse, I took this opportunity to explain how nursing had developed and become specialized over the last century. I went on to explain that nurse midwives are highly trained heath care professionals who closely assess and monitor their patients. I also explained that nurse midwives have lower rates of episiotomies, cesarean births, and epidural anesthesia. In addition, if there is ever a concern about the mother's or baby's health, midwives will not hesitate to consult with or refer the patient to an obstetrician. Nurses, I informed the group, aren't subordinate to physicians. Rather, they have complementary and interdependent roles. They work in different niches and serve different functions, with the goal of improving the health of all people. If nurses and doctors don't work together, I told them, patients die. Finally, I explained the different educational tracks nurses can follow and told them about advanced certification for RNs. The dinner guests were surprised to learn that some nurses have their doctoral degree and conduct research.

The guy remained argumentative. "How could *a nurse* safely monitor a laboring woman?" But the rest of the dinner guests began telling their own positive experiences they had had with nurses. One person mentioned how her primary care provider was a nurse practitioner and she liked how thorough she was compared with her previous physician.

I probably didn't change the mind of the opinionated guy. But I did give him and the rest of our Thanksgiving company something to chew on. And I didn't get indigestion because I had defended my profession.

· · ·

ELIZABETH KOZUB, RN, MS, CCRN, CNRN, is a Nurse Clinician in the Neuro Critical Care Unit, Johns Hopkins Hospital in Baltimore, Maryland, a recent graduate from the University of Maryland with a Master's in Community/Public Health Nursing, and is pursuing a Master's in Trauma/Critical Care Nursing.

Remaking the
Power Nurse

Pierre-André Wagner

She darts through the air, her red hair flying. She wears a tight green shirt, a blue miniskirt, and red boots and carries a thermometer. She looks like Superman's twin sister. She is the Power Nurse. In 2001, she became a symbol of the emancipation of nurses in Switzerland. Her story, the story of her impossible mission, begins in 2001. But let us begin, well, at the beginning.

The year 2001 was also when the Swiss Nurses Association (SNA) hired me as its lawyer. I had passed the bar exam in my home province of Berne fourteen years before. Discovering feminist jurisprudence in Canada in the course of my graduate studies felt like Columbus setting foot on Hispaniola—at that time, gender studies were a dirty word for Swiss lawyers and academics. After my graduation from Toronto's York University, I clerked at the Swiss Supreme Court for a couple of years. *This* was as if Columbus had had to go back to some decrepit hacienda in the midst of the Castilian desert. I decided to dump my job at the Court and do something smart for a change: I went to nursing school—and loved it. Still, the law kept fascinating me, and I went on doing research on my own, until, six years into my career as a neurosurgical nurse, I became the SNA's nurse lawyer.

I had a theory: Each and every problem nurses are confronted with is more or less directly due to the fact that nursing is what lawyers here call a "female-identified" profession. My theory has passed many a reality check since.

The discrimination of nurses and nursing takes many different shapes. The biggest problems were unequal pay and the legal status of the profession. According to Swiss law, nursing was not an autonomous profession, and nurses were legally defined as assisting physicians in their work. Swiss law defines nurses as health professionals who act and who are only allowed to act on a physician's prescription.

At the SNA, we were convinced that nothing would ever change for the better as long as this law was on the books. With the help of a conservative member of Parliament (who liked nurses and whose wife was a nurse), we decided to start an attack in the federal parliament and ask for autonomy for nurses in Switzerland. We knew that we would need the support of the conservative majority. Surprising many of our supporters, we entrusted the motion to amend the health insurance statute to a member of the fairly right-wing national-conservative party.

We also knew that we needed the support of the public if we were to succeed. To the disbelief of many long-time members of our association, we hired a high-profile public relations firm to design a campaign that would convince the public that nursing was able to stand on its own. The firm submitted several ideas to us, and one of them was the Power Nurse. We loved the fact that they used an iconic image and applied it to a profession that people usually think of as passive and docile.

The Power Nurse was born and soon ready to take off.

Many nurses loved her—many hated her. Many hated us—their association—for doing this to them. They were shocked, but what shocked them was exactly what filled others with enthusiasm. The diversity of our profession was made obvious by the multiplicity of reactions to the Power Nurse: the conservative faction was appalled by her immodesty; the post-feminist faction lambasted the use of allegedly sexist imagery; and the vast majority just loved her. Thousands of nurses who occasionally wear tight shirts, miniskirts, and boots—not to work of course—and thousands of nurses who don't, understood that the Power Nurse was not meant to represent *a nurse*. She was a tongue-in-cheek way of symbolizing what we cherish about our profession: its modernity, self-consciousness, and self-assurance.

The media loved her. For quite a long time, the Swiss nurses as well as their association had been pretty much media-averse, content to work in the shadow of front-page politics—to do good and shut up. As for the public, they had been content to admire nurses almost above any other profession, without having to bother to understand what exactly they were admiring them for.

In the 1990s, as the neoliberal ideology and the agenda of rationing reached the health sector, nurses had become aware that their mission—and their livelihood—were in danger. Many began to grasp the relationship between their working conditions and patient safety and outcomes. They got political and their association had to follow suit. Both nurses and their association realized how important it was to go public and air their concerns. But they soon had to acknowledge the tenacity of the public's old-fashioned, angelic, good-girl image of nurses. In this context, the Power Nurse came as a liberating shock. She broke the mold; she busted open the doors of the golden cage. As it turned out, the journalists had avidly been waiting for her, and they relished giving her a platform. She appeared on TV and in the newspapers and shouted: Look at me; here I am; look at what I can do! Would you believe it?!

The politicians loved her. They shook their heads in disbelief, but here she was: It turned out the kind handmaiden would not just stand there waiting for orders but had a voice and would use it to say intelligent things in an intelligible way. As the Chamber of Representatives (like the United States House of Representatives) convened, hundreds of nurses in Nurse Power T-shirts rallied on Parliament Square and lo: the motion to grant the nursing profession autonomy was passed. It passed, quite literally, because the national-conservative party's representatives decided to all go to the restroom. This is a parliamentary trick used when politicians are afraid to vote for a bill and are also afraid to vote against it. Because one of their members had put forth the bill, they couldn't vote against it. But they could not bear to vote for it. With them out of the chambers, we needed a much smaller majority, which we got.

Even though the legislation passed the Chamber it did not pass the Senate. The heated discussion it generated gave politicians a new appreciation and understanding of nursing, which has helped us a great deal. They knew they had to talk with nurses not just talk at them. For the nurses of Switzerland, the world would never again be the same. With the Power Nurse, they had crossed a line and there would be no turning back.

• • •

PIERRE-ANDRÉ WAGNER, RN, LLM, is Chief Legal Officer, Swiss Nurses Association.

Health Policy from Nurses' Point of View

Yuko Kanamori

My background is a little unorthodox. I am from Japan, where I went to nursing school and got my RN license. Soon after I graduated, I moved to the United States and went to college in Georgia to study sociology. Living in Georgia was, not surprisingly, totally different from living in Japan. When I got there, I thought I'd study nursing again. But then I wondered how I could care for patients in a foreign culture without understanding that culture. Moreover, I found out I didn't need to go nursing school again to be an RN in the United States because I already had a bachelor's degree in nursing. I decided to study sociology to learn more about U.S. culture.

After graduating from college with a bachelor's degree in sociology, I moved to San Francisco to work as a research assistant in a job unrelated to either nursing or health care. Because I wanted to do something relating to patient advocacy, nursing education, or health policy, I decided to look for a new job and found a nonprofit organization in Menlo Park, California, whose mission was to contribute to human health. The organization was funded by a Japanese organization and was staffed with medical doctors, businesspeople, and clinical researchers, who were all male.

The job I applied for was that of executive secretary. This is not what I wanted to do, but I thought, "You know what, who knows where opportunities are? This organization is unique, and their mission is broad . . . maybe someday I could have my own project and be more than just an executive secretary."

Fortunately, I got this job and did indeed start working as an executive secretary. I was the only nurse in the group and increasingly felt that the organization—whose mission was to enhance health—needed to include a nursing perspective. Others seemed to appreciate my perspective as well.

I got the chance to inject nursing into their consciousness when my boss, a Japanese physician, asked me if I had any new ideas for a conference that could bring together Americans and Japanese. Without thinking about the organizational and professional politics involved in mounting a conference and after consulting with some experts in nursing, I proposed my conference theme: "health care system reform from a nursing perspective."

At this time, in 2007, the United States was in the middle of a presidential campaign, and candidates such as Senator Hillary Clinton were talking about health care reform. Added to this, Michael Moore's movie *SiCKO* was capturing public attention. I wanted to provide a forum to discuss health care systems from the nursing perspective and to help educate more U.S. nurses about other countries' health care systems and their problems.

My first challenge was to convince the board members of my organization. Remember, I was the only nurse in a group of mostly men, many of whom were physicians from Japan. In Japan, nurses don't usually get involved in politics. (Of course, the Japan Nursing Federation focuses on health policy. But Japanese nurses focus more on bedside care and patient care than health policy such as health care reform.) Some nurses would come from Japan to attend the conference, and some of them said they had no idea why nurses needed to know or talk about health care system reform. They did not believe this was part of a nurse's job.

When I talked to my MD boss about my project, he echoed their sentiments: "I don't know why nurses need to talk about the health care system." We had many meetings about my idea, and then I realized I could not convince him and others in the group without enlisting help. I went to nursing experts at the University of California, San Francisco. Because many professors there are famous in Japan, I knew their support would help. Then I paused and thought, who am I to approach famous scholars such as Patricia Benner and William Holzemer? I was surprised when they answered my e-mails and even more surprised when they met with me and my boss and told him how important it was to consider health care system reform from a nursing point of view.

Although my boss okayed the conference, I had to do the bulk of the work—advertising, setting up the conference site, negotiating with speakers, registration—to make it happen. That didn't matter because close to two hundred nurses—from Japan and the United States—attended. Speakers came from England, Canada, Japan, and, of course, the United States.

Choosing the speakers wasn't easy, and some of the choices proved political and controversial. For example, I had no idea that there was bad blood between the California Nurses Association (CNA) and the American Nurses Association (ANA). Many people at UCSF, for example, were hostile to the CNA because the union had left the ANA in the 1990s—something I learned about in the middle of my stint as a conference planner. Once I became aware of this old wound, I really wanted them to sit at the same table. I was able to make that happen, I think, because I was from Japan. I was neutral and did not belong to either association or side with either party. Maybe they all thought that because I was Japanese, I just didn't know what I was doing, and they went along with it because of that.

Just as I had no idea about the political controversies involved, I also had little idea how to advertise the conference. So I just did it. I called hospitals. Sometimes they called me back. Sometimes they didn't. Sometimes they understood my English. Sometimes it was hard for me to make myself clear.

On the day of the conference, seeing those two hundred nurses and nursing students there was a thrill. I was physically exhausted because I hadn't slept for a week, but mentally I was so happy and honored to be this project manager.

For me this was a beginning. In Japan, I was told that nurses didn't need to know about health care policy. After forcing my company to include nurses in a health care policy conference, I had to force myself to become familiar with the terrain. Now, I'm a student in the health policy program at UCSF School of Nursing. If you had told me I'd be doing this when I was a nursing student in Japan, I'd have said you were crazy.

· · ·

YUKO KANAMORI, RN, got her nursing degree from Gunma University in Japan, earned a bachelor's degree in sociology from Georgia Southwestern State University, has worked as a nursing program development manager and executive secretary at a nonprofit organization in California, and currently is studying health policy at University of California San Francisco School of Nursing.

Maybe We Should Be Bragging

Guðrún Aðalsteinsdóttir

Five of my friends—three RNs, one LPN, and one laboratory technician—and I were playing bridge at my house in Reykjavik, Iceland, recently. I'd been looking forward to the evening. But somehow I just couldn't concentrate. I wanted to talk about what had happened to me that day—I had saved a patient during a potentially fatal emergency—but as a nurse, I'd been socialized not to talk about the good things I have done at work. These experiences are supposed to be just another part of the workday, and to say "I just saved a human life" might make it appear that I was bragging.

I was startled out of my thoughts when my friend Mæja shouted "four hearts" one more time, and Herdis curled her brows. I had to say something, so I just blurted it out, "I saved a human life today!"

My friends stared at me and then demanded to hear the whole story. So with some relief, I told them.

I am an RN with over thirty years' experience, and I work on a nursing unit at a geriatric institution that provides patients with skilled nursing care and long-term care. We have twenty patients who require a great deal of nursing care and over fifty older individuals who more or less can take care of themselves. I was on a morning shift this day, at my post at eight o'clock and, as usual, I didn't know what the day would bring. Even though the days can sometimes seem alike, some are easier and even entertaining, while some are challenging and require me to draw on and expand my bank of experience.

As this particular day went by, I attended my duties, along with two other nurses, two LPNs, and one nursing assistant. About the time we would normally take a coffee break, we were sitting at our first-floor nurses' station, charting and doing administrative work. Suddenly, an in-house phone rang in my pocket. I answered.

"Come right now upstairs to the second floor into the coffee room!" a terrified person shouted into the phone and then hung up without any explanation.

Something was very wrong. I called the other nurse, and we sprinted upstairs. What we found was a group of elderly residents sitting at the coffee table while staff hovered over a white-haired resident in her wheelchair. She was unconscious, her lips blue with not a sign of breathing. The other residents had discontinued drinking their coffee and looked terrified at the scene at hand.

"She choked on a donut," said the LPN. "We slapped her back and did the Heimlich maneuver, without success."

I heard someone else say, "She is dead."

At this moment, my experience and good training from my time on the emergency unit kicked in. I grabbed the wheelchair, the LPN supported the woman's head, and, as we ran with her to a place where there was more room to maneuver, I shouted: "Bring the Ambu bag, oxygen, and call an ambulance."

They jumped into action. The nurse grabbed the bag, someone came with oxygen, and another staff member called for the ambulance. I realized that something needed to be done instantly. The woman was suffocating in front of us. I knew what I needed to do although I had never done it myself. Years before I had been impressed by the performance of an anesthesiologist at the emergency unit during a similar situation. I'd rehearsed the incident in my mind just in case. I knew there was no time to wait for the ambulance. The woman had only a few minutes left, if that.

I grabbed the laryngoscope and Magill forceps from the emergency supplies and asked the LPN to position the woman. We tilted her head back; I slid the laryngoscope alongside her tongue and illuminated her larynx. There it was—the piece of food that was lodged in her larynx. I slid the Magill forceps alongside the laryngoscope and tried to capture the offending morsel. I got part of it on the first try and repeated the process to remove all of the food. Next I gave her plenty of oxygen with the Ambu bag, a device that manually forces air into the lungs.

Seconds later, though it seemed longer, we heard her snarl and then gasp for air. It's hard to convey how happy we were at that moment. Slowly, she started to breathe. By the time the ambulance with the physician arrived, she was starting to regain consciousness. She was transferred to a hospital but came back to us a few days later, fully recovered.

My friends clapped and hugged me. I think they were even a bit impressed. I know we're not taught to talk about all the important things we do—even among ourselves. But I think we should talk more. Maybe we should even be bragging!

· · ·

GUðRÚN AðALSTEINSDÓTTIR, RN, has been a practicing nurse since graduating in 1974 from the Icelandic Nursing School, in Reykjavík, Iceland, where she continues to live and work.

Finessing the Chairman of the Board

Carol Blount

I was seventy-four when this happened and had been practicing nursing for fifty-two years. For many of those years, I did not talk to non-nurses about nursing work. I, like many other nurses of my era, was taught not to brag about our work. By the time I reached my early seventies, however, I had read many books and had enough experience, and I'd decided it was time to change—time to speak out.

My chance to do that came at a Christmas party given by my financial adviser in December 2005. I stood with a group of businessmen dressed in coat and tie and women in bright red dresses. We watched a boy's choir sing Christmas carols. A Christmas tree twinkled with white lights. Waiters carried trays of tiny cheese biscuits and shrimp skewered with red and green toothpicks. People smiled and sipped their Christmas punch.

I joined a couple I knew who were talking with a man I did not know. We had a brief introduction. The couple suddenly announced they had to leave, so I was left with my new acquaintance. We exchanged "and, what do you do?" questions. I stated I was a nurse in home care and asked him if he knew what nurses did in home care. He said "only in general," so I gave him a brief description of my job.

I explained that the nurse acts as case manager, coordinating all the care the patient receives at home. She follows the doctor's discharge orders, performing skilled nursing assessments and technical procedures. She monitors patient progress and reports change in status to the patient's physician. If appropriate, she teaches the patient and family wound care, diabetic management, medication teaching, and home safety. A fall at home can mean rehospitalization, a setback for the patient, and increased hospital costs. Early recognition of a problem can prevent repeat hospitalizations for symptoms that can be managed in the home. We discussed how home care's role had expanded in the past few years as the length of patients' hospital stays had decreased.

I then asked him what he did in the hospital. His answer was, "I do fund raising." Recalling a recent fund-raising hospital brochure I had received in the mail, I said: "Well, you won't get one penny from me until you change your brochure; it so angered me that I threw it in the wastebasket."

The man looked surprised and asked, "Why, what's wrong with it?"

I answered, "It contains pictures only of doctors, one fold-out after another, giving their name, specialty, and a short write-up. I turned the brochure over, expecting to see pictures of nurses and other members of the hospital team explaining their work. But, there on the other side were more doctors, smiling and looking confident, and most of them are men."

The man was listening. I was not shy; here was my chance to speak up to a hospital person in fund raising and tell him what I thought. So, I continued.

"Where is the emphasis on teamwork that the hospital proudly refers to? The public needs to learn about the many professional members of the team, and their contribution to patient care. People will be taken care of by nurses in the hospital, and they need to see their faces in your brochure. This brochure does none of these things."

My companion continued to listen attentively, receptive to what I was saying. We both forgot the people around us at the party and continued engrossed in our conversation. Then I ventured, "What exactly do you do in fund raising?"

"I'm the chairman of the board at the hospital," he answered and told me his name.

I blinked, gulped, and, when I recovered, said, "I'm happy to meet you."

To my surprise, he said, "I will go right home tonight and research this; I know who is responsible for writing these pamphlets."

I realized I had been fortunate to meet such a receptive chairman of the board (COB). I had explained to him what nurses do and the importance of sharing this with the public. He had listened to me, and I hoped he would follow up on our conversation. We bid each other goodnight and Merry Christmas.

In a few days, I received a phone call from him. He said he had voiced my concerns and that he hoped in the future I would see a new brochure with more focus on the hospital staff. I thanked him for his follow-through and said I would look forward to seeing a new brochure.

I didn't imagine that we'd see each other again, but the world is full of surprises. That spring I received a coveted invitation to the annual employee dinner sent to staff members who have worked at the hospital for five years or more. As I entered the hotel for the party, I hoped I'd see the COB. I had recently learned that a prominent nursing and patient advocate was coming to our hospital on Nurses' Day to lecture. I wanted to invite him to attend. When I saw him in a cluster of people near the bar, I walked up to reintroduce myself and plunged right in: "Do you remember me? I'm Carol Blount, the nurse who did not like your hospital fund-raising brochure."

"Indeed I do," returned the chairman flashing a pleasant smile.

This was encouraging, so I continued on. "I have come to invite you to the Nurses' Day lecture in May at the hospital. We are having a distinguished speaker who will explore nursing issues in hospitals and in general and suggest possible solutions. I think you should come."

I waited what seemed like an eternity but was probably just a minute, before he answered: "I would be delighted to come, please send me a memo with the date and time and check with my secretary to make sure I am free. Also, I would like you to invite the president of the hospital and tell him that I said he should come." The thought of doing this bold deed gave me pause, but I couldn't stop now, so I agreed.

Then he said, "And one more thing, I will come on one condition."

With apprehension I asked, "And what is that?"

"That you will sit right beside me at the lecture."

Relieved, I said I would be delighted.

At the dinner table, my friends were curious about our conversation. "What did you say to the COB?"

"I invited him to our Nurses' Day lecture, and I think he's coming. He wants me to invite the president, too!"

"Really, I can't believe you did that," said one nurse.

"Why not?" I asked. "He needs to hear about nursing issues and some of the challenges we face. What better day than Nurses' Day?"

And indeed, when that day in May rolled around, he was in attendance and I was there to greet him. I had invited the president of the hospital as requested, but, due to a scheduling conflict, he was unable to attend. The conference room soon filled with nurses. We sat in the front row.

The COB sat quietly listening and took notes during the lecture. When it ended, the speaker asked if anyone had questions. To my surprise, the COB raised his hand and asked the first question. When the question period ended, several nurses came up and spoke to the COB. They said they were pleased he had come. When asked if he enjoyed the lecture he said, "Yes, I've learned a lot about nursing, and I'll share some of these ideas with the board."

I received numerous e-mails from nurses after the lecture with positive comments such as: "I view my work differently now, I respect what I do for patients" and "I speak differently with the doctors now; I have more confidence in myself." One nurse asked me how I got the COB to come to the lecture. I said it was simple: I just asked him.

This positive chain of events occurred because, at a Christmas party, I voiced my opinion. My good fortune was that the "fund raiser" I spoke with just happened to be the COB.

New brochures had been printed with broader coverage of the hospital team. An avenue for improved exchange of ideas had opened between nursing and hospital administration. I hoped there would be many more Nurses' Days like this one. A piece of advice to nurses: Attend more parties, speak up; it's just possible you could be speaking to the COB!

· · ·

CAROL BLOUNT, RN, BSN, has worked in many settings since receiving her RN degree in 1954 from Boston Children's Hospital and BSN in 1980 from the College of New Jersey, including twenty-five years as a home care nurse; she currently maintains a part-time practice providing health screening and wellness teaching in Princeton, New Jersey.

Called to Duty at 30,000 Feet

Ann Converso

I worked as an RN for more than thirty years, before re-tiring this year from the Veterans Affairs Western New York Health Care System in Buffalo, New York, where I was a medical-surgical and intravenous (IV) therapy nurse. I now serve as president of my national union, the United American Nurses, AFL-CIO (UAN). In our union, we often use the slogan: "Every patient deserves a registered nurse." By that we mean, every patient and family should have an RN available to make critical assessments, observe changes in condition, and advocate for the needs of the patient. Lives are at risk when RNs are not accessible—either in the hospital or in any other setting where health may be at risk.

Nurses will always rise to the occasion and offer their expertise, whether on duty or off. Every nurse has had the experience, in daily life, of being sought out for health care advice. Often it's a friend or relative just wanting information or reassurance about a minor problem. Sometimes, however, you are asked to step in and deliver life-saving care to a complete stranger on a street corner or at the scene of an accident.

I got the latter kind of call to duty on a recent plane trip from Buffalo to Phoenix. Well into the flight, 30,000 feet up, a flight attendant got on the loudspeaker, looking for a nurse on board. Usually such emergency queries begin with a canvas of any available MDs and, if no one answers, they next ask for an RN. This time, the flight attendant ignored the usual sequence for requests, asking anxiously: "If you are a doctor *or* a nurse, please ring your call button."

From the tone of her voice, the situation sounded serious, so I immediately got out of my seat and hurried up the aisle to where another, worried-looking flight attendant stood. She was leaning over a man in his twenties, dressed in jeans and a T-shirt, with a military-style haircut. He was in the aisle seat; a young woman next to him was asking for help and saying he wasn't responding. (We learned later he was a military police officer on leave and traveling to Arizona.) I quickly assessed our sick passenger and determined that he needed immediate intervention to stabilize his condition. I tried to take his pulse, which was barely perceptible. He was clearly fevered, in distress, and breathing with great difficulty.

I was soon joined by another passenger on the flight, a female doctor, who also volunteered to help. While the flight crew debated the merits of making an emergency landing with the pilot, I asked the doctor for an angiocatheter so I could start an IV. As she hesitated to select the right item from the medical kit, I was reminded that not all doctors are medical doctors, and not all physicians insert IVs as part of their day-to-day work. It was clear that she didn't know how to do this and that I did. She said that she would do whatever she could to assist, but I was clearly in charge. As I started the IV, she inserted the IV tubing in the IV bag and began opening other equipment that might be needed. After I put in the IV, we ran normal saline wide open, Ambu bagged the young soldier (pushing air into his lungs with a hand-held device), and tried to stimulate him verbally and physically by talking to him as loudly as possible.

About twenty minutes later, after receiving a liter of fluid and having air forced into his lungs, the young man's condition stabilized. He began to be responsive; I could feel a better pulse and hear a blood pressure. He started talking with us, we gave him some orange juice, and he came back to his normal status.

I was able to return to my seat, where one of the flight attendants offered me a drink. She told me the story of her husband's near-death experience, due to a serious motorcycle accident. "It was nurses in the ICU who saved his life," she said, "not the doctors. It was the nurses who were there at his bedside every minute, every day of his sixteen-day stay in the ICU."

How rarely, I thought, is that same real-life scene shown in TV shows, films, or newspapers. Instead, the media spotlight always seems to be on the doctors, even though in actual hospitals (and in other emergency situations), the doctor is not always the only "expert" on the scene and every member of the health care team has a valuable role to play.

On my return trip to Buffalo from Phoenix a few days later, I was surprised to see my emergency patient—now doing much better—board the same flight I was on, accompanied by his fiancée. Just to be on the safe side, they joked, perhaps they should sit near me?

Fortunately, there was no call for any further assistance—for the soldier or anyone else. But I knew there was at least one passenger aboard who would certainly now agree: "Every patient deserves an RN!"

· · ·

ANN CONVERSO, RN, worked for over thirty years as an acute medical/surgical and IV therapy nurse at the VA Western New York Healthcare System at Buffalo. She currently serves as president of the United American Nurses and sits on the AFL-CIO Executive Council, the only nurse to hold a seat there.

Part 7
APPLIED RESEARCH

I'll never forget the first story I did on nursing research. I pitched the piece to a health science editor at the *Boston Globe*. "This would make a great story," I said. "It really highlights the value of nursing research."

Her response was: "Nursing *what*?"

Like so many members of the public, this journalism expert had no idea that nurses do research. She was equally surprised to discover that nurses play a major role in conducting, implementing, and monitoring medical research. I was a lot like her when I first started writing about nursing. Programmed by shows like *Marcus Welby, M.D.* and the health science sections of newspapers, it never occurred to me that nurses did research. I, too, was surprised to learn they did and even more surprised to learn the role nurses play in what we think of as medical research. Nursing researchers like my good friend Kathy Dracup quickly taught me about the breadth and depth of the research nurses conduct. I've been learning from nurse researchers for years.

The nurses who speak in this section demonstrate the wide scope of nursing involvement in advancing our knowledge of wellness and illness, aging, and human vulnerability as well as of the problems nurses have doing their work. To do this, they may have to buck physicians who cling to the idea that "the doctor knows best" (even when he or she isn't the "principal investigator" involved in a grant-funded research project). And they simultaneously need the backing of nurse managers and chief nursing officers, who are uniquely positioned to provide access and support for the kind of research that actually improves patient care. They may even take on entire industries or encourage their colleagues to view research with a critical eye.

These stories also help us understand the connection between research and much-needed organizational change. As the nurses here explain, research laurels aren't just a leg up the academic ladder for them personally. Their work can help make our health care system more cost-effective and humane. It can also provide nurses in practice with the intellectual ammunition they need to construct an environment capable of attracting, rather than repelling, competent providers of hands-on care.

Nurse PI on a Clinical Trial

Kathleen Dracup

Many of the problems patients have today can be addressed and answered only by teams of clinicians. No one discipline can solve the complex problems of very sick patients. This is as true in the research setting as it is in the clinical setting. A clinical problem is always multidimensional, and every discipline brings a special expertise and way of looking at the problem. For example, if a patient is on medication, it's helpful to have a pharmacist involved in the research. Patients have limitations in functional status, so we need physical therapists. Patients often have dietary issues, so it's helpful to have someone who knows about nutrition. Nurses know what modifications patients and families have to make to deal with their problems and what the clinical symptoms are and how to manage them. Physicians are educated about pathophysiology and how to diagnose and treat disease.

For many years I have done research to test different solutions to patients' clinical problems with teams of doctors, nurses, physical therapists, pharmacists, and others.

To be successful, we need to recognize that everybody brings valuable expertise to the table. But unfortunately, health care is hierarchical. At the top of the medical hierarchy, there are surgeons and subspecialists. Family practitioners and pediatricians often feel they are at the bottom. As you go down the hierarchy, traditional stereotypes are alive and well. Hospital culture is militaristic—with titles like "chief medical officers" and terms like "doctors' orders." This hierarchy can get in the way of the kind of shared authority and open communication that we now know support patient safety and good care. As a nurse scientist, you have to be prepared to confront this kind of hierarchy when you engage in research.

A case in point is a study I did to help patients with advanced heart disease while they waited for a heart transplant. These patients are often tired and have limited exercise capacity. So as we help them remain active, we encourage them to increase their exercise. Physical activity is important because not exercising at all can decrease patients' ability to cope with the transplant situation. Daily exercise, furthermore, can serve as an antidote to depression, decrease the fatigue patients feel, and improve quality of life.

To understand the role of exercise in this patient population, I conducted a study with a group of physicians, nutritionists, and exercise physiologists to see if we could increase exercise capacity by having patients do a carefully supervised home exercise program. This was a clinical trial conducted with 175 patients, half of them randomized to an exercise program and the others, the control group, asked to do only normal activities but not to exercise regularly. I was the person who wrote the grant and was therefore the principal investigator (PI). About half of the research team was composed of physicians, and the rest were from other disciplines.

In this case, as in so many others, I was reminded of the historical traditions nurse scientists have inherited. In decades past, nurses were expected to collect the data on research teams but were never the PI. Although that has changed dramatically, even as PI you still confront vestiges of the "doctors write the orders, doctors are in charge" mentality that exists in hospitals. Since this study was conducted in an outpatient clinic attached to a hospital transplant program, a lot of those same traditions still applied, despite the fact that I was the PI.

Even though I ran the research meetings each week, I could sense these historical tensions. They came to a head when the patients in the exercise group began dying at a much higher rate than the patients in the control group. Although none of the patients in the exercise group died while exercising, nine patients in the exercise group died and only three patients in the control group died. That was a 300 percent difference and was alarming to everyone.

The question was: Should we stop the trial?

The physician who was the director of the clinic and the primary physician on the team felt strongly that we should stop the trial and publish a paper stating that "exercise is bad for you" if you are a patient in this situation. He thought that would make a wonderful and interesting paper. I believed that the numbers were so small that these deaths—distressing as they were—could just be random. I argued that we should not do what was more dramatic but not good science and instead should continue the trial. We consulted with the funders and the monitors—the Data Safety Monitoring Board. We had a long meeting with this board, and they agreed with me and said we should continue the trial. At the end of the trial, the numbers of deaths in each group were the same; there were as many deaths in the exercise group as there were in the control group. It turned out that it was not exercise but rather the disease that led to patient deaths in the exercise group. Patients with advanced heart failure have very high mortality, and the people who participated in the study did not exceed the expected rate.

When the research team debated these findings, it was clear that the physician, who was identified as the coprincipal investigator on the research team, was used to analyzing the situation, making a diagnosis—or in this case identifying and labeling a problem—and then having his analysis become reality. If I had been a physician PI, the dynamic would have been very different. Although there was a lot of communication and mutual respect, we had several heated meetings because my physician colleague believed strongly that we should stop the trial and perhaps, although he never said it, equally strongly that he should be listened to and obeyed. I had to strongly disagree on the basis of the science and equally strongly articulate my position. I did, and we found out something that has proved to be very important to transforming the quality of life for patients waiting for a heart transplant. In the end, we discovered that exercise is not harmful for patients with advanced heart failure, as had been previously thought by many clinicians, and can even be beneficial.

• • •

KATHLEEN DRACUP, RN, DNSc, Dean and Professor, School of Nursing, University of California, San Francisco, has published widely on cardiovascular disease and interdisciplinary collaboration and has served as a co- or principal investigator on numerous clinical trials designed to test interventions for patients with heart disease.

The Need for Nurse Evaluators

Teresa Moreno-Casbas

As chief of nursing research at the national level in Spain, I struggled long and hard to get nursing research funded. Finally, because we refused to give up and maneuvered behind the scenes, we have had some success.

Here's what we were up against.

To get a research project funded in Spain, a proposal has to go through the Spanish equivalent of the U.S. National Institutes of Health (NIH), the Instituto de Salud Carlos Tercero, and be evaluated by a panel of evaluators. Unfortunately, until 2004, the people who were chosen to be evaluators on the institute's initial evaluation panels as well as on its final decision-making panel were primarily male physicians. At first, these physicians didn't want to fund nursing research, which they didn't take seriously, at all. After much struggle, they finally agreed that maybe nursing research was a legitimate field and should be funded at the national level but insisted that they should be the principal investigators (PIs) on all nursing proposals.

Why? Because they actually knew something about nursing research? No! It was because, they insisted, the only way to ensure proposals would be taken seriously and eventually funded was to have a physician as the PI. Without a physician PI, even one who had no significant knowledge of nursing issues and research questions, physician-evaluators would not grant the funding and physicians who were chiefs in hospitals wouldn't give nurses research access. The line was, "I, the physician, will be the PI and take care of you, the nurse."

I knew that we had no chance of conducting nursing research with nurse PIs if we did not change the composition of the evaluators on panels. This would be the only way that nurse researchers would be truly reviewed by their peers. In Spain, peer reviewers are selected via a database. The problem was that not enough nurses' names were included in this database. So potential nurse peer reviewers were invisible to the system. To change this, we needed to include the names of potential nurse reviewers. My opportunity to do this appeared in a surprising way. It turned out that the database was extremely difficult for anyone to navigate. So I offered to help fix the database. While I was doing that, I said that I would add the names of "some" nurses.

And I did exactly what I promised. I rearranged the database to make it more user-friendly, and I included the names of some nurses. Now we have nurses on the panels and on the groups that make the final decisions based on the evaluations of those panels. This has given us the ability to get nursing research funded without a physician PI.

Oh, and did I mention that when I was helping to reconfigure the database, I included the names of one hundred nurses? That's "some," isn't it?

• • •

Teresa Moreno-Casbas, RN, MSc, PhD, head of the Nursing Research Coordination and Development Unit at the Carlos III Health Institute, has published widely on the topic of nursing research, knowledge transfer, and elderly people and has served as a principal investigator and coinvestigator on numerous national and European research projects.

Research and Nursing-Home Reform

Charlene Harrington

For over thirty years, I've been researching and writing about the nursing home industry and working for improvements in the quality of nursing home care. It's been a long journey that began in 1975, when Jerry Brown was governor of California. I had just received my a PhD in sociology and higher education from the University of California, Berkeley. With that and my nursing background, I got a job working for the California Department of Health Services and was later placed in charge of the agency that regulated all health care facilities.

That was my introduction to the nursing home industry. What I discovered was the extent to which nursing home residents were suffering because there were almost no regulations governing nursing homes at that time. This wasn't only true in California but all over the United States. In fact, just as I was working on regulatory and enforcement issues in California, the U.S. Senate began holding hearings about the poor quality of care in nursing homes across the nation.

To remedy these problems in the state, we developed stricter regulation and oversight and went after some of the poorest-performing nursing homes. We were determined to force some of the worst homes out of business or to seek more responsible ownership of them. This was not a pleasant or easy process, nor did it earn me any popularity with the nursing home industry. For example, one of the homes in California we had to shut down was a four-hundred-bed nursing home whose patients were dehydrated, had pressure ulcers, and even died due to poor-quality care. The owner was from New York, and dealing with the home was very confrontational. I had to send inspectors into the home around the clock, and we had attorneys and investigators build a case to force the owner out. Because we couldn't find a new owner, and the building itself had serious problems, we eventually had to shut it down.

Again, this was not an easy decision. A lot of the families and advocacy groups didn't want the patients moved out because they were worried about where they would go. Even though the placement problem was resolved with enough thought and time, it was stressful for the residents, families, and staff. To this day, the nursing home owners and administrators in California remember that this was the first time anyone had taken them on and actually enforced the regulations. These enforcement efforts were later used to make recommendations for a change in federal survey and enforcement activities recommended by the Institute of Medicine in 1986 and for the nursing home reform legislation passed by Congress in 1987.

When I left state government to take a position at the University of California, San Francisco (UCSF), School of Nursing, I continued my work on nursing home reform—this time as a researcher on nursing home quality, structure, and regulation—especially staffing. Staffing, I now think, is the most important issue that affects nursing home quality. Unfortunately, in spite of years of effort, federal law on nursing home staffing is still weak. The law stipulates only that there must be one—that's only one—RN on duty eight hours a day, seven days a week, and an additional licensed nurse on the evening shift and on the night shift regardless of the number of residents in a facility. States can go beyond the federal requirement, but that minimal, national standard has been the law since the Nursing Home Reform Act was passed in 1987.

To help the U.S. nursing home reform movement, I've conducted research that attempts to build the evidence necessary to improve regulations and staffing. There is an active movement for nursing home reform in the United States, and advocates lobby state legislatures and Congress to improve conditions for nursing home residents. As they speak to policymakers, the public, and the news media, these advocates need more than anecdotal stories describing some terrible thing that happened to someone's mother or father in a substandard nursing home. Of course, we need those accounts, but we also need a statistical profile of the industry. This kind of research can be used by groups such as the National Citizens Coalition for Nursing Home Reform (NCCNHR) that take the kind of data I have generated and distribute it to Congress, state legislatures, and the media.

To reform nursing homes, I have also used research to make recommendations to the Clinton administration on the design and development of the Medicare Nursing Home Compare website (www.medicare.gov/NHCompare) to help consumers get needed information that will help them make choices about nursing homes. Such websites also serve another purpose, which is to motivate nursing homes to improve quality so that facilities will get better reports. I also designed and developed a nursing home report card website in California for the California Healthcare Foundation in 2002. The website provides information on staffing, turnover, complaints, deficiencies, quality measures, and cost information. The data are used to rate nursing homes and have rated all the nursing homes in California. Later, in 2004, we started rating California home health agencies and hospice programs. We update the website every quarter and now we're trying to make the website more understandable to consumers.

In December 2008, the Centers for Medicare and Medicaid Services (CMS) began its five-star rating system on www.medicare.gov/NHCompare. The website in California was used in the design of the Nursing Home Compare rating system.

When it comes to nursing homes, research is not an abstract exercise designed to brush up a tenure file or sit on a dusty shelf. It's a spur to action. The fact is, it is difficult to get Congress and state legislatures to act on the basis of anecdotes alone. Even with research, getting them to act sometimes seems like a Sisyphean task. But without the research data, nursing home residents would still be where they were when I began working on the issue in the 1970s.

• • •

CHARLENE HARRINGTON, PhD, RN, is Professor Emeritus of Sociology and Nursing at the University of California, San Francisco, and is the Principal Investigator and Director of the National Center for Personal Assistance Services at UCSF, a project funded by the National Institute for Disability and Rehabilitation Research (2008–12).

How Nurses Make It Work

Kathryn Lothschuetz Montgomery

In the late 1980s, when I was chief nursing officer at a research hospital, an exciting research study for the treatment of cancer was being studied in a phase 1 human clinical trial. Researchers were studying the impact of a biological modifier as a potential cancer treatment. The major focus of phase 1 clinical trials is to determine toxicity and efficacy. In this phase 1 clinical trial, lymphocytes—cells from patients' blood—were withdrawn and treated so when they were reinfused, the treated lymphocytes in combination with specialized drugs would act to destroy the cancer cells. The intervention had had extensive study using laboratory models and was now ready to be introduced for the first human trial.

The family and patients on this initial study experienced a sense of hope and determination because their advanced cancer and prognosis offered only one outcome: death. The principal investigator (PI) of the study—an oncologist—had years of scientific effort and study invested in this trial and held high expectations for this new approach for cancer treatment. The physicians and nurses providing the patients' clinical care were given a lengthy briefing on both the scientific study and the patient's clinical needs.

After the patients began treatment, the nurses involved in the study—all of whom had extensive experience in clinical research care and experimental studies—began to identify major psychological symptoms in some of the patients. At first, physicians dismissed the symptoms as stress or the progress of the disease. It soon became apparent, however, that a trend in these symptoms had emerged only in the patients who had received the intervention. In some patients, the response was quite dramatic. They were becoming agitated and at times violent. They were suffering from hallucinations and becoming paranoid. Some believed their nurse was going to hurt them. Some were disoriented, unable to recognize family members. These were clearly not symptoms of the kind of stress a patient like this would routinely experience. Nurses were concerned for both the patients' and family members' safety as well as their own.

Because of this, the primary nurse brought her findings to the clinical rounds and reviewed each case with extensive detail. The physician PI and the clinical care physician dismissed the nurse's observations and report of trends. You could almost hear what the physicians were thinking as they responded to the nurses' concerns. They seemed to believe that psychological behavioral symptoms were not part of this study intervention and that the patients were predisposed to this behavior because they were under stress as a result of their cancer and poor prognosis.

The primary nurse persisted and sought validation from her nurse colleagues and family members. I was consulted on how to manage the difficult and unprecedented clinical situation and provide direction on how to obtain the appropriate resources to manage the patients and family. They sought the help of the nurse psychiatric liaison consultant—an advanced practice nurse who has expertise in the management of psychiatric symptoms, disruptive behavior, and grief responses of patients and family members, especially in medical-surgical settings.

The primary nurse and her nurse colleagues continued to see increased behavior changes. It was apparent to the nurses that the behavior was not based in a stress reaction, and the fear that families felt was increasing. The psychiatric liaison nurse and primary care nurse worked through an approach to prevent harm and ease the symptoms that included structuring the environment by reducing stimuli, removing glass and sharp objects, and having a consistent and trusted nurse with the patient and family at all times. In addition, the nurses pursued the help of staff psychiatrists. Together they explored the biological linkage between the study intervention and select neurotransmitter physiology of the brain and functioning that resulted in the behavioral changes and increasing risk of disruptive and violent behavior.

After many attempts to engage the cancer clinical care physician in dialogue about the behavioral changes and the need for treatment to resolve them, the primary nurse, psychiatric liaison nurse, and psychiatrists presented their own clinical rounds and hypothesis on why these symptoms were emerging to the PI and research team. Nurses and psychiatrists finally convinced the PI that this aggressive immunological intervention was the basis for this behavioral change. The PI joined forces with the nurses and psychiatrists in the development of a preassessment guide to facilitate early identification of patients at greater risk of the side effects. He also worked with them to prepare the patients and family for what they might experience with these symptoms. The group, now working together, agreed to make sure that any patients in this study received every kind of help possible to minimize the behavioral symptoms and provide a sense of safety for the patient, family, and nursing staff. They were committed to do anything that would allay the concerns of the family when they witnessed this dramatic change in the personality and behavior of their loved one.

Patients and family members contributed to the development of a plan that included extra observational status by the nurses, psychiatric drug intervention, and safety measures in the patient's room.

The outcome of breaking through the isolation and arrogance of a highly scientific, driven PI and team resulted in a specialized care protocol for this patient population and opened the door to a new research direction that continues today. Without the clinical expertise and leadership of this primary nurse and her colleagues in identifying this cluster of behavior symptoms, the immunological and neuropsychiatric health interface in the human body would not have seen its current advances.

It happens at times that a brilliant physician is wrong. To make matters worse, the mistake or problem is ignored because a hunch or trend that a nurse identifies is dismissed.

Fortunately in this case, I was committed to helping steep the nurses in this organization in professional esteem and leadership, and we all had the capacity to pull together the collective expertise of other disciplines to make a convincing case. We continued to make that case with persistence, interpersonal and interprofessional competency, and knowledge. We were thus able to help the first group of patients and families in this clinical trial, ensure the value of the cancer discovery, and open the door to further research on the immunological and neuropsychiatric interplay that continues today in both original lines of research.

. . .

KATHRYN LOTHSCHUETZ MONTGOMERY, PhD, RN, is Associate Dean, University of Maryland School of Nursing; she has had many years of executive experience in research and academic organizations, is former Chief Nurse at Clinical Center NIH, and is a USPHS Rear Admiral Retired.

Teamwork through Research

Lena Sharp

Before 2005, oncology patients in Stockholm received their care at two different university hospitals—one in the north and one in the south part of the city. All that changed when the two hospitals merged into one—the Karolinska University Hospital. Mergers are always tough, and this one was no exception. Despite being in different parts of a very large city, the two radiotherapy (RT) units were supposed to function as one. How could we do this, staff wondered—particularly when no one was happy about the merger?

Although we knew that the merger could eliminate long wait times for patients, we also recognized that patients would only be able to benefit if we, the clinical staff, were able to overcome some serious divisions. There were, for example, some significant problems between doctors and the nurses—who in Sweden have advanced, specialized nursing education and provide radiotherapy, which is not the case in most other countries. There were also problems between doctors and medical physicists and biomedical engineers. These problems preexisted the merger. Now, added to all this, we had tensions between nurses in the two sites.

After a year of settling into the new organization, the nursing management of the RT unit, consisting of five head nurses (of which I am one), two clinical nurse educators, and a nurse manager, started to discuss what we could do to improve collaboration across both RT sites. We wanted to improve patient care and team functioning as well as empower nurses in their contacts with the other professional groups with whom they work closely (i.e., nurse assistants, medical engineers, physicists, and physicians).

We began to recognize that most problems we dealt with were related to communication issues. Not surprising, given what we now know about error's connection to communication and teamwork, we also uncovered a substantial number of reported errors that were attributed to inadequate communication. Hierarchy and rivalry among professional groups was a major problem. When we tried to solve these conflicts, our attempts seemed to cause even more conflicts and hurt feelings. Nurses, physicians, and physicists all believed that no one listened to them and that the other professional groups didn't appreciate their knowledge, skills, and responsibilities.

It was clear that we needed to do more than episodically attempt to resolve problems. We needed to implement a systematic and long-lasting educational program in communication for the RT nurses and nurse assistants. I contacted a professor in nursing at the Karolinska Institute, Carol Tishelman, with whom we had previously worked, and we collaborated on developing a proposal for funding a communication training program. The Swedish Cancer Society granted us enough funding to carry out most parts of our planned education project, with the working name "Communicate More." We also solicited the input and support of physicians and physicists during the early stages of planning. This wasn't easy because many of us believed that it would be difficult to motivate physicians and physicists to be involved in the project. One of the big surprises was our discovery that we were totally wrong. After some initial suspicion, it turned out that there was no problem in engaging these groups, although hierarchy among professionals was an even greater issue than we had imagined.

Our next task was to find experts in communication to help us develop our ideas for the content. We formed a project group combining nursing clinicians, teaching faculty, and academics.

To get a better understanding of the communication issues in our organization, we began by holding six focus group discussions (FGDs) with representatives for all the professional groups at both RT sites. This included FGDs with staff from units other than RT (e.g., oncology inpatient wards, chemotherapy units, and outpatient clinics). One FGD included representatives from various patient organizations with experience of RT at our department. A nurse researcher with no other contact with our organization led the FGDs.

These groups revealed that we had even more problems with hierarchical issues than we expected. For instance, we learned that to avoid disturbing physicians on lunch breaks, some RT nurses didn't follow the treatment guidelines. Some physicians said—out loud—that things had been better when the nurses had shorter, less specialized education. They suggested that RNs should focus only on their technical tasks rather than, as they do today, on providing advanced cancer nursing care. The FGDs also highlighted problems between the two RT sites and between different nursing teams within the RT units. Nurses in one unit thought they were more competent and skilled than nurses in the other, who were described as more "touchy-feely" and less knowledgeable. One unit was referred to as a factory, the other as more humane. Obviously, these issues and concerns not only damaged morale but also had the potential to seriously compromise patient safety.

During the planning process, the head of the oncology department changed twice, and the nurse manager and head of staff for RT also changed. Two of the five head nurses changed (twice) as had one of the clinical nurse educators. All this made the information and implementation phase more difficult. But we persisted nonetheless.

We felt it was important to hold the education program using people close to and involved in the RT department to make sure we could follow up and implement changes adequately.

To get proper skills to perform the education program, we hired outside consultants to help us develop a train-the-trainer course. After that we worked on planning the first course that these trained trainers would lead.

Our current goal is to train 130 RT nurses—from both sites—in groups of ten. During one session of the course, representatives of other professions will also be invited to speak. We will then have a workshop on hospital hierarchies and discuss ways that other high-risk industries—such as commercial aviation—have done trainings to enhance safety and increase teamwork. We have just started the third out of five or six planned courses for nurses and also arranged the follow-up sessions for course one and two. We are also planning a special course in patient safety and team communication for the managers for all professional groups involved.

When we recognized we had a problem, we could have done what nurses have so often done in the past—ignored it and soldiered on. We decided not to do that. Instead, we decided to get the knowledge to do something positive to correct the problem. Even though we are in the beginning stages of that process, communication, morale, and patient care are already better as a result.

• • •

LENA SHARP, RN, PhD, specialist in cancer care, is Head Nurse of the Radiotherapy unit at Karolinska University Hospital, Stockholm, Sweden, and is the president of the Swedish Cancer Nurses' Society.

Keep Asking Questions

Sean Clarke

In my career as a researcher and professor, I try to teach my students, as well as suggest to my peers and the public, that we always need to keep an open mind and to look beyond the surface when thinking about health care and nursing. This is particularly true when there are inconsistencies in the information we're seeing, and especially when the questions being asked are unpopular and risky. Today, one often hears experts argue that some risk factor or variable is or is not important for patients, that a way of educating nurses or organizing nursing services is right or wrong, or that a treatment approach is good or bad. It's easy to accept such statements as gospel truth without much reflection, especially when they confirm deeply cherished beliefs.

What I've learned as a researcher is that the only way we can improve patient care and nurses' working lives is by devoting energy and efforts to research and then respecting a principle known as the self-correcting nature of science. In other words, if we apply our research skills in good faith, make efforts to build on past knowledge, and open our work to scrutiny by others, over time, we will better understand the factors that affect patients' outcomes and change patterns of care and health care delivery for the better. Single studies, and even small series of studies that lead us toward a specific conclusion, prove nothing. Extensive scrutiny and the test of time are needed to be confident in a conclusion, especially one that's popular with certain audiences in our profession or outside of it. All researchers—me included—and all studies—including my own—are open to question.

A commitment to caution and reflection in talking about research, as well as an aversion to oversimplification, has lost me a popularity contest or two over the years.

I worked for a number of years as a trainee, and later as a collaborator and administrator, in a well-known nursing research center in the United States. In our group, we published several papers that garnered much attention. These papers touched on some of the "big" questions within the profession: Are nurse staffing levels in hospitals connected with anything of real importance to patients or the health care system? Are there any links between the educational profile of a hospital's nursing staff and that hospital's outcomes? Are nurses generally unhappy with their work because they're complainers—or are they mostly unhappy about specific aspects of their working conditions? Are all hospitals created equal as places for nurses to work and for patients to receive care?

Sometimes it was easy to come forward with our results and the papers were heralded by (almost) all. And sometimes it was not easy to come forward at all. For instance, when our results suggested that Pennsylvania hospitals with higher proportions of baccalaureate-prepared nurses on the front lines of care showed lower risk-adjusted mortality rates, some people were very upset. They felt as if we were undermining the position of community-college graduates in the profession—who, like it or not, represent and will continue to represent a large share of those who work as registered nurses in the United States. Others committed to university education for nurses were driven to overstate the conclusions that could be drawn from this work. Despite my commitment to university-level education (full disclosure: I've taught for over a decade in three different bachelor's programs), I felt a need to write an article in my own voice clarifying my take on our findings, and was joined by a national leader in the community college nursing movement in doing so. But careful writing and sensitivity only went so far.

Discussing research findings is not an easy task, and I always try to correct people's misinterpretations of my work and others' research data. The misreadings come in a variety of forms, but the reality is that there's just no way to draw iron-clad conclusions from the kind of data researchers are usually forced to use. This is because hospitals, nurses, patients, or clinics are different from each other, and the patients treated across different hospitals are going to vary in important ways as well, and we can never take everything of relevance into account and rule out all competing explanations. Nonetheless, while there are limitations in the most common types of research we're able to conduct, we can learn (and have learned) much from working with information collected for other purposes and gathered through our observations and careful questions to providers and consumers of health care.

It's obvious to me, and starting to be clear from an increasing mass of studies, that nurses and patients are better off in hospitals where CEOs and CNOs recognize that nurses are knowledge workers and manage them accordingly. In these hospitals, nurses' observations and opinions about clinical care and the environments in which they practice are given heavy weight in decision making and as a result, high-quality care is never an accident: It is deliberately nurtured. But the evidence that justifies this conclusion is not necessarily as "hard" as we'd like it to be, and saying that we've "proven" a case, or that positive outcomes are "caused by" this or that factor, is probably going too far. What we have done is found results "suggestive" of certain phenomena being linked to specific types of outcomes.

That's why it doesn't usually surprise me when work I've done is greeted with a shrug or a snort by those outside the profession. But it's sometimes shocking to me when nursing colleagues argue that results that they don't like are biased or insist on a conclusion that the data may actually contradict. In our profession, especially in the circles occupied by highly credentialed nurses, people tend to believe they have "the" answer and that "if only" the forces in the health care system would listen to their suggestions and not hold us back so much, society would be better off. The reality is that we have many interest groups within the profession, and a history of not only being held back by outside forces but of turning on each other. I'll go out on a limb and say that I've been shocked by how scientifically illiterate even very educated people in the profession can be. And also how politically naïve they sometimes are. Guess what? No one's opinions, certainly not in the upper reaches of government or in the health care industry, are ever going to be reversed by one or a handful of specific study results—and certainly not by interpretations of specific papers that anyone with a basic understanding of research methods could easily challenge.

I've been amazed at how downright nasty some efforts to squelch open discussion on critical decisions about the profession's direction can be. And that antiscientific and antidemocratic impulses usually come from both poles of most struggles within nursing—from both the "pro" and the "con" sides of the eternal entry-to-practice education debate, the benefits of Magnet hospitals, and on and on, and on. It's as if we've decided that scrutinizing the "guts" of a study to determine whether or not its conclusions hold water is only necessary when research is used to support a position we don't like.

The longer I conduct research, the more I am convinced that "truth" is complicated, subtle, and sometimes painful—but that we and our patients are always better off when we have research data in hand and when we take intellectual risks (and when necessary, personal ones) to send them out in the world so that they can stimulate discussion.

Ideas with long pedigrees as well as newfangled ones must always be tested—that's the essence of evidence-based practice and management. The nurse on the front lines of care as well as the researcher must question, value the questioning as an activity in and of itself, and protect those willing to question when doing so seems dangerous. When the conversations get emotional, I always remind myself that working with any data, however imperfect, and being tough-minded in interpreting them, is *always* better than blind faith in untested assumptions. There are a few non-negotiables in nursing: putting patients' interests first, being purposeful and thoughtful in caring or helping others provide nursing care, and working to improve over time. Pretty much everything else in nursing and other human services work should be open to vigorous inquiry—the tougher the better. Our feelings can stand up to the questioning and so can the profession.

· · ·

SEAN CLARKE, RN, PhD, FAAN, is the RBC Chair in Cardiovascular Nursing Research at the University of Toronto and the University Health Network hospital system in Toronto, Canada, and he holds adjunct and visiting appointments at universities in Montreal, Philadelphia and Dublin.

No More Martys

Jane Lipscomb

Early in 2006, Jonathan Rosenblum, a community organizer with the Service Employees International Union (SEIU) Local
1199 Northwest in Seattle, Washington, contacted me about the issue
of violence in the workplace. He was familiar with research that the
University of Maryland Work and Health Research Center had done
with the New York State Public Employee Federation (PEF) around
the safety hazards to New York State community mental health workers. He requested our assistance with a similar situation in Washington State. During a subsequent call, we learned of the tragic death of
a SEIU Local 1199 Northwest member, Marty Smith, a County Desig-
nated Mental Health Professional (CDMHP). Mr. Smith was mur-
dered in November 2005 while making a home visit. The mother of
a young mentally ill man called about her son's behavior. He was acting erratically and was off his medication, and Smith went to the home
and the son stabbed him to death.

Following Marty's death, SEIU conducted a survey of its members
and began an effort to pass legislation that would improve safety for
the mental health workforce, the community at large, and ultimately,
individuals with mental illness. Now SEIU wanted us to do fieldwork
to understand the hazard and make recommendations to the legislature. My colleagues, Kate McPhaul and Matt London, and I worked
with the union to design a field study. We spent four days in Washington meeting with mental health managers, state mental health and
safety experts, labor leadership, and consumer representatives and
conducting structured focus groups of community health workers
representing four distinct regions in northwest Washington State.

During this fieldwork we met dozens of experienced, courageous,
caring, professional mental health providers and other advocates for
the mentally ill who have dedicated their lives to caring for this se-
verely underserved segment of the population. These professionals

199

face many challenges as they try to provide care to the mentally ill. Like Marty Smith, they work with individuals who have complex needs. Mentally ill people are not inherently dangerous or violent. In fact, those who are under competent and consistent care are not at increased risk for hurting themselves or others. Tragically, however, many mentally ill patients are not given the help and resources to deal effectively with their own illness. This means that health care workers like Marty Smith often walk into homes where they encounter agitated, even dangerous, patients. Because their work is woefully underfunded, these workers all too often go into homes by themselves and without backup. What happened to Marty Smith is an inevitable result of this kind of underfunding and neglect of both the mentally ill and the workers who try to care for them.

Rather than stigmatizing the mentally ill, the conclusion of many providers and workers in this field with whom we spoke is that more attention and resources must be devoted to the care of the mentally ill for the safety of the consumer, the public, and the workforce alike.

In September of 2006, SEIU organized a press conference that featured the release of our report and recommendations. At the press conference, the bill's sponsor Rep. Tami Green (D), Ms. Smith (Marty's widow), and my nurse colleague Kate McPhaul, who took the lead in writing our report, spoke about Marty, the proposed bill, and our fieldwork report and recommendations. All three local news networks and the *Seattle Times* covered the press conference.

Our recommendation, based on the findings from the visit as well as the experience of the researchers, national best practices, and the federal Occupational Safety and Health Administration (OSHA) Guidelines for the Prevention of Workplace Violence in Healthcare and Social Service Workers (1996/2003), included two major thrusts. First, we argued for continued legislative and policy efforts to increase funding for community mental health. The ultimate objective is, of course, improving the quality of patient services through reducing the size of the caseload mental health workers must shoulder. We also argued strongly that, in high-risk cases such as this one, or when there is some question about removing a child from the home, the state should mandate that mental health workers be accompanied by a second person when they visit a home.

The second focus of our recommendations was the creation of a state commission that would evaluate the magnitude of the problem of violence against such health care workers. This commission would be mandated to identify further interventions to protect workers, including the development of a training curriculum that focused on skills for preventing violence when making home visits and certifying trainers.

In May 2007, the Marty Smith bill (Senate Bill 556) became state law after it passed both houses of the state legislature unanimously. Sponsored by Rep. Tami Green, mental health RN and SEIU member, the act will provide annual safety training for all community mental health workers; ensure that CDMHPs and crisis intervention workers will not have to go out alone on high-risk home visits; and ensure better access to case files so these workers know when they're going into a situation that might be dangerous. The Marty Smith law is the strongest law in our country governing the safety of mental health workers who do high-risk outreach visits in the community.

· · ·

JANE LIPSCOMB, RN, PhD, FAAN, is Professor and Director, Work and Health Research Center, University of Maryland Baltimore School of Nursing.

Taking On Conventional Wisdom

Thóra B. Hafsteinsdóttir

Being a nurse researcher isn't always easy. One of the things we do is evaluate the effectiveness of contemporary practice and treatments. If our results demonstrate that current approaches aren't effective, some people—like the bedside nurses who have mastered a particular technique or treatment or other professionals who are working with nurses—may be unhappy with our results and aren't shy about conveying their displeasure.

That's just what happened when I, as a stroke researcher in the Netherlands, was asked to evaluate what is known as neurodevelopmental treatment (NDT), a rehabilitation approach for stroke patients that had just been introduced on the neurological and neurosurgical wards of the University Medical Center in Utrecht. Nurses on both wards had to attend educational courses about the treatment and also underwent rigorous on-the-job training. They had finally become comfortable with the approach, when, to their surprise, a professor of neurology suddenly asked the nurses whether NDT was really effective. People thought it was, but no one really knew.

That's how I came into the picture. I was asked to conduct a study measuring the effects of NDT on various patient outcomes. After carefully considering all the possibilities, we came up with a non-randomized comparative design, with a large group of patients, where the effects of NDT interventions on functional status (mobility and activities of daily living [ADLs]), shoulder pain, depression, and quality of life would be measured. The study was conducted in twelve hospitals. In six hospitals, nurses and physical therapists used the NDT, and in six hospitals they did not.

After two years of data collection and analysis we found that NDT made no difference to patient outcomes. In fact, even the traditional approach to stroke rehabilitation care as usual or conventional nursing, which did not include NDT, was more effective than NDT. Patients who were cared for with NDT were not more able to care for themselves, did not have better functional status, did not have less shoulder pain, were not less depressed, and did not have better quality of life. When I relayed these messages to the nursing community, suggesting that nurses carefully consider other ways of caring for patients with stroke, my results exploded like a bomb.

I started receiving e-mails with questions and comments (not all of them friendly) from nurses and other professionals concerning the study. I did interviews with nursing papers about the findings. Even one of the morning papers published an article on the study, with a headline—completely inaccurate—quoting me as saying that "rehabilitation does not work."

Despite my best attempts to nuance the discussion, large groups of nurses and physical therapists who had used the NDT for years were very angered by the news. I knew the evidence supported my conclusions, as did other Dutch researchers within the physical therapy and rehabilitation science arenas. Unfortunately, they never talked as publicly and critically as I had. So there I was, feeling isolated and attacked and wondering how I could continue my work in the midst of this firestorm.

I was, however, determined to continue with what I considered important work for patients and had a meeting with the nurses on the wards participating in the study. The first question they asked me was, "How are we supposed to care for the patients if the NDT does not work? No other rehabilitation approach has been worked out." I told them that it might be possible to develop a clinical practice guideline focusing on rehabilitation nursing of patients with stroke. I got a green light from the management teams where I was working. We set up a project with a multidisciplinary team of professional experts (including professors of nursing science, physiotherapy, and rehabilitation medicine), forming a steering group along with stakeholders, agencies for health care, and representatives of professional nursing organizations in the Netherlands, and we held meetings on a regular basis to develop the guideline. The working group included ten nurses and researchers from the Netherlands and Iceland. In the process of the guideline development, all the recommendations were reviewed by a group of thirty-three expert professionals, made up of nurses, physical therapists (PTs), occupational therapists, clinical neuropsychologists, dieticians, speech language therapists, rehabilitation physicians, sexologists, and patients, who carefully judged the draft version of the guideline in two sets of rounds.

After more than three years of careful work, we came up with an evidence-based guideline for the rehabilitation of stroke patients. Our guideline includes eleven chapters on various topics such as mobility, ADLs, falls, nutrition, swallowing problems, dehydration, cognitive problems, communication problems, depression, sexuality, and education of patient and relatives. Each chapter contains recommendations that nurses can use in their daily care of patients with stroke.

You might think this was the end of the story. After all, we had a guideline that contained a thorough literature review and clearly documented and tested approaches. But there were still battles to come. This time the battle cry wasn't raised by nurses but by some of the other professionals who reviewed the various recommendations. When, for example, a neuropsychologist read the guideline suggesting that nurses, who are after all the ones who care for stroke patients 24/7, be responsible for screening for cognitive status, emotional status and depression, and swallowing function, she questioned whether nurses (i.e., "just nurses") could possibly be held responsible for conducting such screening and threatened to report this to her union or her association. I explained that we were not suggesting that nurses conduct full assessment of cognitive status. Nurses, however, were perfectly capable of using the available recommended screening instruments, such as the Mini Mental Status Examination, intended for the first screening, and they had been doing this for decades.

I also received a letter from a speech language therapist who didn't want to see a guideline that formally asked nurses to screen patients' swallowing. We also had some discussion with physical therapists (PTs), who questioned some of the recommendations that focused on nurses' assisting patients with exercise and mobility. Traditionally nurses aren't the ones who help patients with exercise. Nurses do range-of-motion and breathing exercises, but when it comes to ADLs, there's a line in the sand with nursing on one side and PTs on the other. Our evidence showed that it is crucial to train patients to relearn ADLs in their daily life on the wards and not only to train them in the exercise room away from the ward. Walking the patient on the floor is as effective as (but more efficient than) letting the patient exercise walking on a treadmill. I therefore explained to the worried PT why we included the recommendation that nurses assist patients with training walking on the ward.

Finally, after much *sturm und drang* (storm and stress) we now have a Dutch evidence-based Clinical Nursing Rehabilitation Stroke-Guideline (CNRS-guideline), which includes a total of 211 recommendations that nurses can use in the daily care of patients with stroke. When, in January 2009, we held a symposium on the guideline, more than two hundred nurses attended, and we received many positive e-mails about the guideline. Nurses from various groups have joined forces to collaborate on setting up educational programs and preparing for future implementation of the new CNRS-guideline. Even though some people may think that the hardest parts of developing an evidence-based guideline are conducting the literature review, collecting and analyzing the data, and writing up the results, I believe that the toughest part is getting real people in real workplaces to change behavior on the ward. That's a challenge that never ends.

· · ·

Thóra B. Hafsteinsdóttir, RN PhD, is Associate Professor, University Medical Center Utrecht and Research Centre for Innovations in Healthcare, University of Applied Sciences Utrecht, the Netherlands, as well as an adjunct associate professor at the Faculty of Nursing, University of Iceland.

Part 8
STICKING TOGETHER

Despite the inspiring stories of individual patient advocacy told in section 5, there are times when one person acting alone can't make enough of a difference. To advocate successfully, there are times when RNs must also act together—a reality of the workplace world that not enough nursing schools seem to explain to their students prior to graduation. I find that nurses are repeatedly exhorted to be individual patient advocates but that the concept of collective advocacy is poorly developed. This failure to explain, or sometimes even acknowledge, the limits of individual advocacy can lead nurses to become demoralized. Determined to act to protect their patients, nurses leave school brimming with enthusiasm and then discover the stark realities of the workplace. When they realize that they can't advocate effectively on their own, they may blame themselves for this problem. Sometimes, they may also blame other nurses or nursing culture itself.

Fortunately, many nurses quickly recognize that you can't fight or change a big institution if you don't work collectively. This is, after all, the lesson of nursing's history. By joining together over the last two centuries, nurses have transformed their own practice and the workings of the modern health care system. In the age of Florence Nightingale, they created order out of the chaos of the nineteenth-century European hospital. In North America, they founded and built three-quarters of the hospitals that enabled new settlers to survive the perils of new world. Here and abroad, they were responsible for developing major nursing schools and organizations ranging from the American Nurses Association to the International Council of Nurses. Nurses have formed unions and many other professional organizations. They have also worked in alliances with other groups to effect change.

Today, RN collective bargaining organizations represent the vast majority of nurses in the industrialized world and a growing percentage of nurses in the United States (nearly 20 percent). These unions and other nursing organizations have won workplace improvements that benefit both RNs and their patients, while becoming much more influential players in public policy debates about the future of health care. In tough fights about staffing ratios, from California to Australia, they've even taken on the "Terminator" himself—Arnold Schwarzenegger—who learned, the hard way, that Hollywood-born governors aren't the only ones with a little muscle. In many settings and struggles, by sticking together, groups of nurses have prevailed against the odds. And a lot of times, they've had fun doing it.

Winning Recognition of Nursing Expertise

Edie Brous

Traditionally, nurses have been considered simply physician extenders. It was assumed that doctors were the only health care providers with sufficient expertise and knowledge to "captain the ship." All other providers were secondary and subservient to the physician. Consequently, in a negligence or malpractice lawsuit, physicians were considered the obvious persons to serve as expert witnesses.

Physician expert witnesses testified in all health care cases, regardless of the provider being sued. If a nurse was sued, it was a physician who would be considered the expert. It was the physician who would translate nursing practice for a lay jury. It was a physician who would determine the standard of nursing practice required in the particular matter. And it was the physician who would testify that in his or her expert opinion, the nurse did or did not depart from those nursing standards of practice.

While no court would consider allowing a nonphysician to provide expert testimony for or against a physician, the courts had no trouble allowing physicians to testify as experts for and against nurses. The underlying assumption seemed to be that, although nurses do not know everything about medicine, physicians do know everything about nursing. Simply being a physician rendered the physician an expert on all facets of patient care. Nursing was subordinate to and under the direction of the doctor; therefore, doctors could render expert opinions on *nursing* care. Hmmm.

The American Association of Nurse Attorneys (TAANA) was in the process of conducting research on which states allow physicians to testify as experts for other health care professionals when an actual lawsuit regarding just this issue was en route to the Illinois Supreme Court. In *Sullivan v. Edward Hospital* (209 Ill.2d 100 [2004]), a hospital was sued when a seventy-four-year-old hospitalized man fell to the floor, sustaining a subdural hematoma. The plaintiff's expert witness, Dr. William Barnhart, was a physician who testified that the nurse was negligent. This "expert" in nursing had not attended nursing school, had never taken nursing boards, and had never practiced nursing.

Most likely, the good doctor also never conducted nursing research, never subscribed to nursing journals, never sat on a nursing committee, had zero experience interviewing, supervising, educating, or disciplining nurses, never contributed to a nursing textbook, and never wrote any nursing policies and procedures. Part of the "expert" testimony included his opinion that the "nurse missed the diagnosis of delirium completely." Hmmm. This "expert" in nursing clearly did not even know the scope of practice for nurses, as he was unaware that nurses do not diagnose.

TAANA submitted a brief to the court supplemented by multiple statutory authorities and scholarly publications. The nurse attorneys argued that nurses and only nurses are qualified to render expert testimony and opinions regarding nursing. Opponents argued anachronistically that, "physicians can do anything a nurse can do" and are therefore qualified as nursing experts. After all, they work with nurses every day and observe nursing practice enough to be familiar with nursing standards of practice. Well, I observe newscasters every day, but that does not make me a media expert.

There are sixty nursing boards in this country, and none of them permits a person to practice nursing without a license. A physician cannot practice nursing unless he or she has attended an accredited nursing program and successfully passed the licensing examination. MD or no MD, this same "expert" in nursing would not be legally allowed to practice nursing. TAANA argued that nursing is not "some lesser appendage of the medical profession."

In its research, TAANA had discovered that only physical therapists were allowed to testify as to physical therapy standards of care. Only chiropractors were allowed to render expert opinions on the standard of care for a chiropractor. Only audiologists, psychologists, or podiatrists were allowed to offer testimony regarding the standards of practice for their fields. And certainly, only physicians were permitted to serve as expert witnesses for medicine. Yet nursing practice was still considered to be within the purview of a physician's expertise.

Nurse attorneys took this on. They conducted research, prepared and submitted a brief, and traveled to hear oral arguments. On February 5, 2004, the Illinois Supreme Court filed its opinion, extensively citing the TAANA brief and supplemental authorities:

> TAANA argues that Dr. Barnhart should not be permitted to offer expert testimony against nurse Lewis based on his observation of nurses. We agree. By enacting the Nursing and Advanced Practice Nursing Act . . . the legislature has set forth a unique licensing and regulatory scheme for the nursing profession. As TAANA observes, under the nursing act, a person with a medical degree, who is licensed to practice medicine, would not meet the qualification for licensure as a registered nurse, nor would that person be competent to sit for the nursing license examination, unless that person completed an accredited program in nursing. (*Sullivan v. Edward Hospital*, 209 Ill.2d 100, 2004, p. 122)

In other words, the only expert competent to testify as to the standard of care for nurses is a nurse. The American Association of Nurse Attorneys said

> it is unlikely that any physician, unless he/she has completed a nursing program and has practiced as a nurse, can offer competent, reliable expert opinion on these nursing standards. It is unjust and ill advised to allow the medical profession to continue to offer expert, opinion evidence on the standards of care for nurses. This practice undermines the ability of the profession to set its own standards or to define its scope of practice. A nurse could be found liable for failing to perform to the physician's standard when, in fact, he/she was acting within the scope of his/her own license as determined by professional organizations and state nurse practice acts. At the very least, this practice invites jury confusion and inconsistent verdicts. TAANA believes it is time to clarify the law and to accord to the profession of nursing the recognition, autonomy and respect given to every other health care profession in the United States. The nursing profession and only the nursing profession has the right, duty and responsibility to determine the scope and nature of nursing practice including the standard of care for nurses. (TAANA position paper, June 27, 2007, Experts on Nursing)

It is TAANA's position that the only expert competent to testify as to the standard of care for *nurses* is a nurse.

And now, because of the efforts, skill, education, expertise, and advocacy of *nurse* attorneys, so said the court!

Don't you just love it when you win?

• • •

EDIE BROUS, RN Esq., is a nurse attorney specializing in medical malpractice defense litigation, professional licensure representation, and nursing advocacy.

A Union Just for Nurses

Massimo Ribetto

It was the summer of 2000. I had been working as a nurse for just three months, at the regional hospital in Bolzano, Italy, when, for the first time, I took part in a meeting called by unions that represented nurses along with many other workers. (In Italy, large industrial unions—allied with political parties—represent multiple categories of workers. Traditionally nurses were not in unions of nurses—or even unions of other health care workers—but were in politically allied unions with journalists, steelworkers, or actors.) Faced with the lack of nursing personnel—what politicians were referring to as a "nursing emergency"—that plagued the hospitals of the province at that time, the politicians decided to set aside extra funding to increase the salary of nurses. This, they hoped, would motivate a profession in crisis.

During the meeting, the participating unions had to decide on the criteria that would be used to apportion and distribute funding among the various groups of nursing personnel. What impressed me about that meeting was that the union representatives—probably because of their ignorance of the nursing profession—were unable to provide leadership about the issues under discussion. None of them was a nurse. But, more important, the union organizations they represented included among their members workers employed in all the categories of work done in a hospital. Perhaps because of this diverse membership, their policy had always been to try and make everybody happy without regard to differences among the various types of workers and professionals.

That meeting in the summer of 2000 ended, and no one was happy that no significant decisions had been made to address the nursing crisis. The nurses argued among themselves about how to distribute the funds earmarked for them. The union representatives, who were supposed to manage the meeting, were not able to reach any conclusions. In subsequent months the nurses did get a salary raise, but they were not the only ones. In order not to disappoint anyone, the unions channeled the money earmarked to deal with the "nursing emergency" to the other groups of hospital workers as well. This significantly reduced the raise earmarked for nurses. This undermined attempts to lighten the workload of the nurses, which was due to short staffing. This episode opened my eyes to the problems of Italian unions and nursing in the health sector in Italy.

After this meeting, several nurses, including myself, began to wonder about the possibility of forming some kind of new union—a union that, unlike the ones we knew, could better represent the interests of nurses. At the end of the same year, 2000, I and two other colleagues from my floor came across something called Nursing Up.

What was Nursing Up? It was a new union, founded three years earlier in Rome by a nurse. Its goal was to represent nurses in collective bargaining and to protect them as they exercised their profession. Nursing Up is a union that represents a specific category (trade) of workers and that finds its strength in the profound knowledge of the profession and its professionals. Although it is a union of nurses at the service of nurses, its knowledge and competence in the field of health care allows it to come up with health care strategies and policies that are useful to the broader community.

In October 2000 my colleagues and I contacted the highest leadership level of Nursing Up and our colleagues in the close-by city of Trento where the union was already known and established. We started recruiting on the floors of the Bolzano hospital, introducing the union to our colleagues and signing them up as members. In subsequent months the number of nurses who decided to join Nursing Up increased dramatically, and within two years we signed up enough numbers to gain representational rights in collective bargaining, on a par with the other union organizations.

All this took place within the span of two years. During that time, we had to work hard and overcome many obstacles to give birth to this new union organization. One major hurdle was overcoming the objections of other Italian unions that—perhaps not surprisingly—strenuously opposed our efforts. These union members didn't simply stand by on the sidelines broadcasting their disdain or disagreement. In some cases, representatives of the other unions in our hospital began to write and distribute flyers encouraging nurses not to join our new union. They tried to discredit us and Nursing Up in every way they could. The larger unions even threatened us. My colleagues and I received personal phone calls telling us not to leave the larger unions. These representatives even claimed that we would lose our jobs if we allied with this new union. Rather than discouraging nurses from believing in the newly born single-category union, these attempts to sabotage our efforts backfired and encouraged more people to join our union.

The greatest obstacle we faced appeared during contract negotiations when the other unions agreed with the administration to raise the threshold of representation from 5 percent to 15 percent. Traditionally, to gain representation in a hospital, 5 percent of nurses had to be union members. But to thwart our efforts, the unions decided that now 15 percent would have to join. This created a one-year delay in reaching recognition of our union's right of representation within the province but was not enough to bar us from participating in the negotiations. In 2003 Nuring Up was officially recognized by the province of Bolzano.

Since then, Nursing Up has grown in numbers and experience. In every major hospital of our autonomous province, we have an office and a group of colleagues working for our union. Over the past few years, we organized two demonstrations and a provincial strike and collected signatures among the population for various petitions in order to gain greater visibility for issues of concern to nurses. For example, we addressed a petition to the local population asking for an increase in nurses' salaries and recognition as a distinct category when negotiating job agreements with the hospital administration. In eight years of activity, we published scores of articles in local papers. We signed four collective bargaining agreements within health care facilities and two contracts for the public employees of the province.

The challenges don't end here; the goals we plan to achieve are many. What makes us most proud and pushes us to do even more is that increasing numbers of nurses are joining our union. We know nurses need help articulating their concerns, and we are there to give it.

• • •

MASSIMO RIBETTO graduated from the University of Verona, has worked in Bolzano, Italy, as a cardiology and oncology nurse, and is a regional coordinator for the Nursing Up union in the Alto Adige region.

We Rained on Their Parade

Judy Sheridan-Gonzalez

In 1987, when changes in financing resulted in increased patient visits in our large Bronx, New York, teaching hospital, our nurses' union contract was reopened. At the time, registered nurses were grossly underpaid across the United States: starting salaries had just crept up to the level of sanitation workers; longevity pay, however, was either nonexistent or capped out at a few hundred dollars annually. Nurses with twenty-five years of experience received little more than a certificate.

Our large teaching hospital in New York City employed many single-parent nurses, forced to work second jobs to pay their rent or mortgage. Facing a critical nursing shortage, the hospital offered a modest increase in starting salary, a strategy in sync with the rest of the League of Voluntary Hospitals, their administrators' coalition. As president of the local bargaining unit, I knew that management needed to increase new-hire salaries to remain competitive in the market—but increasing experience steps would benefit the bulk of nurses in the long and short run, as well as show respect for nursing expertise.

The hospital refused to negotiate. They simply placed their offer on the table, sure that the nurses would never say no to new money. At the same time, they were spending close to half a million dollars on an opening ceremony publicity event on November 22 for a new state-of-the-art building they had just constructed that would substantially expand the medical center's physical plant.

Over the previous year, the administration of the hospital had begun embracing a business model as opposed to their former clinical focus. We had loved our jobs until then, and patients received extraordinary care. Now we were facing the loss of autonomy and professionalism, with patients reduced to "products" based on their reimbursement rates.

217

A small group of nurses, including myself, formed a committee, which strategized around how to win longevity pay and respect for the union and to create a scenario that would empower and politicize the nurses for this and future battles. We discovered the mayor would be present at the opening ceremony for the new building. The hospital had gone to great lengths to bring the mainstream media in, as well as entertainment, performers, and food and prizes for the community. We seized on the idea of having a counterdemonstration across the street the same day.

We organized quietly until the last minute. We had helium balloons in pink and red that said "RNs: an endangered species" and signs reading, "For a party: $450,000; For the nurses: peanuts." We prepared song sheets, chants, thousands of multilingual leaflets, noise makers, banners, signs, and markers. Patients, families, senior citizens, doctors, hospital workers, and all of our nurses mobilized to show up in force. On a cold day in November, we pulled out over one thousand people. We assigned nurses to walk the halls and ask folks on their break to make an appearance when the media showed up. And all the major TV stations were there.

Our demonstration was so spirited that the hospital performers—clowns, stilt-walkers, and all—crossed the street to join *our* party. So did patients, visitors, and the news media. Even the mayor was forced to make a statement. It was a Sunday with no other hot news item that night. The hospital's opening was reduced to providing a backdrop for the nurses' story on every news station!

We saw ourselves interviewed en masse, singing songs, chanting, holding up signs with powerful messages about staffing, patient care, and experience. There was even a clip of an angry hospital administrator chastising an acrobat who joined us, overheard saying, "We're paying you—you're not supposed to be here—these nurses are not with us." We played that clip over a hundred times. The nurses, many new to activism, felt enormously empowered.

The hospital increased their offer the next day, insisting in a written letter to the nurses that this had nothing to do with the previous day's "activities." The nurses were giddy with their newly discovered power. While the money was substantial, management still offered nothing for longevity pay and refused to sit down and negotiate. They made the incredible blunder of publicly stating that studies had shown that after seven years, a nurse's "value" plateaued. Infuriated by this blatant denigration of their experience and expertise, the nurses voted down the money and blitzed the hospital with letters that said, "We will only vote for a settlement that is negotiated with our elected leaders" and signed their missives with their years of experience—most past the "plateau" of presumed mediocrity. There was much colorful commentary regarding the "seven year" studies in conversations and in letters.

By January 1988 we broke the League's boycott of longevity pay via a negotiated settlement and set into motion a campaign to provide similar increases for nurses at our "competitor" hospitals the following year. Nurses, mobilized by our militancy, subsequently engaged in multiple successful campaigns to improve our dismal pension benefits, preserve our flexible scheduling, avoid future givebacks and layoffs, and fight for contract language that protected patients and promoted quality care.

We also established a tradition of pickets and rallies whenever we negotiated successor agreements. Emboldened moments on the picket line, singing and chanting—while managers watch nervously from the sidelines—create a rare feeling of "leveling the playing field," according to many nurses. Occupying the lower-middle tier of rigid hospital hierarchy, nurses may suffer humiliating treatment and unjust discipline on the units. Being out on the streets en masse provides us with the opportunity to see ourselves in a different light. Sometimes, we bring that feeling back inside, cultivating the courage needed to ward off the bullying and punitive actions of the hospital machinery.

The hospital rationalizes our spirited rallies as little more than a show. One administrator commented—to a nurse he characterized as "reasonable"—that the hospital "tolerated" such events as a mechanism for the nurses to "blow off some steam." The nurse replied, "On the contrary. This is just a warm-up."

. . .

JUDY SHERIDAN-GONZALEZ, RN, is president of a large Bronx hospital's local bargaining unit of RNs, represented by the New York State Nurses Association, serves on NYSNA's Board of Directors, is past president of its Delegate Assembly, and is one of the founders of NY Nurses United, an independent pro-democracy caucus of NYSNA.

Protesting on the Red Carpet

Kelly DiGiacomo

When I became a nurse in 1995, it was at the height of the hospital restructuring of that era. I worked in California for a large health care organization in postpartum, newborn nurseries, pediatrics, and then telemetry. At this time nurses were constantly being threatened with layoffs and downsizing. I was so worried about losing my job in the mother-baby unit that I left the main hospital and took a job in our pediatric clinic because, at the time, layoffs were not threatened there. Many nurses were so nervous about the layoffs that they either left the hospital, like me, or left nursing altogether, which didn't help the nursing shortage which had become a serious problem in California as well as nationwide.

In the hospital, the workload was unbearably heavy. There were no nurse-to-patient ratios, so staffing levels varied day to day. You could have as many as eight patients assigned to you. One harrowing night still stands out in my mind. We were very short staffed due to sick calls and vacations. There was no extra staff scheduled. I was working on the postpartum unit and, due to short-staffing, was told I would be caring for fifteen moms and their babies. It was so unsafe. I worked in an isolated back nursery on the night shift. If I had an emergency with an infant, I had to phone up to the front desk for help. Most nights working in post partum, I felt like I was running down the halls, throwing pills at my patients. I dreaded what to do if they asked me a question because I didn't have time to answer them. One night, I got home from work so exhausted that I flopped onto the couch in my uniform and immediately fell asleep. The next day when I woke up, still in my scrubs, I wondered how much longer I could do my job.

Many times I thought about leaving nursing. I was torn between my love of the profession and the craft of nursing and my love of people and for my patients. But these extreme working conditions were just too much. I suffered a severe work-related back injury due to the heavy physical demands of caring for so many patients in a fast-paced setting. I had no life outside of work. I was constantly exhausted when I was with my husband and kids.

I wanted to quit many times, but how could I? I was the sole breadwinner for my family. I had a twelve-year-old daughter and a sixteen-year-old son and a husband that was being treated for leukemia and couldn't work. I was the only one. I couldn't quit. I wondered how many nurses out there were like me? We have families, young children, and maybe a sick family member, and we're going into work and taking care of very sick people under these incredible conditions. And then we have to go home and take care of more sick or vulnerable parents, spouses, or children.

When my husband was at Stanford Hospital undergoing a life-saving bone marrow transplant, I had to drive two hours each way between home and his hospital bed. I found myself dividing my time between work, caring for my children, and trying to care for my husband. It was an unbelievably difficult time, and I could not afford to take any time off from work. Occasionally, when my husband's status was precarious, I could not leave him and had to call into work for a family emergency. One day, I was called into my manager's office and I was reprimanded for "not smiling" enough at work. I could not believe it. I asked if my work was deficient or if there were any complaints against me. My manager said, "No, we have just noticed that you are not smiling enough." My boss was aware that my husband was gravely ill. I felt this was retaliation for my being absent from work even though I was using all of my own earned vacation time. There were no federal laws back then to protect workers for family medical leave such as this.

This treatment by my manager was one of the many reasons why I fought so hard to get safe nurse-to-patient staffing ratios in California and thus better treatment for nurses. I was elated when the legislature finally passed the bill in 1999 and then the governor of California signed it. After the ratios were enacted, work started getting better. I went from caring for eight to ten or more patients on the telemetry unit to caring for no more than five; it was a total transformation. I felt safe. I felt patients were safe.

And then in 2004, right after President Bush was elected for the second term, Arnold Schwarzenegger, who was elected governor of California in 2003 in a special election, suspended the implementation of the ratios. Nurses felt like we'd received a punch in the stomach. And we began to fight all over again.

When Governor Schwarzenegger announced the termination of the ratio phase-in, the California Nurses Association (CNA) began a campaign to put public and political pressure on the governor to rescind the emergency order. We followed him around the state and the country, wherever he went. I went to Boston, New York, Los Angeles, and San Francisco to protest him. I regularly led CNA-organized protests at the capitol in Sacramento against him. We shouted into bullhorns and carried picket signs. This was not an image of nurses that the public or the media was used to! The media, always at these events, publicized that the governor was taking on the nurses, who are in one of the most time-honored and respected professions. It just did not make any sense. He also tried to take on teachers, police officers, and firefighters. I thought, who will be next, nuns?

In December 2004, the governor spoke to ten thousand participants at a women's conference in Long Beach. Nurses were outside picketing, and he stopped his speech to inform his audience to "pay no attention to those voices over there. They are special interests. Special interests don't like me in Sacramento because I kick their butt."

I wasn't at that protest, but I went to another one closer to home. Governor Schwarzenegger was making an appearance at a movie premiere of *Be Cool* with its stars John Travolta and Uma Thurman in Sacramento. As celebrities paraded into a downtown theater on the red carpet, nurses picketed outside with red signs. The CNA was able to get one ticket for one nurse, and I was it. So I went into the movie theater to take my seat. I was dressed in my nurse's uniform, lavender scrubs; I didn't have a purse and wasn't carrying anything other than my ticket, driver's license, and a cell phone. I took a seat near the front of the theater and made a couple of calls while I waited for the governor's arrival.

Suddenly, a plainclothes security officer employed by the governor approached me and asked me to move to the back of the theater. I refused. He asked for my ticket and identification, which I gave him.

He looked at them and at me, gave them back, and again asked me to move. I said no. He left, and I sat back down. A few minutes later, he came back and asked me if I would like to "speak with the governor." I knew that I would not be allowed to talk to the governor, but I said "yes," and I was led to a small room in back of the theater stage. I waited. Soon, a huge highway patrolman (he must have been at least six foot four and I'm only five foot two) came and guarded the only door to this small room. He did not introduce himself, and he made it clear that I was being detained. The governor was nowhere to be seen, but for an hour they interrogated me like I was a terrorist or a criminal. Over and over, they asked for my name, date of birth, Social Security number, who I was with, why I was there. I kept asking if I could leave, and they wouldn't let me. They kept me away from the governor until the movie premiere started and the governor had left the stage.

Finally, they said I could go, but they wouldn't let me back into the theater; they led me down a dark and narrow hallway that had a door that opened to the street behind the theater. I went back outside and joined the nurses picketing in front of the theater. I told my fellow nurses what happened, and the news spread that Schwarzenegger, the bulky bodybuilder, was scared of a tiny California nurse. The story made headlines. In one, he was dubbed "the Paranoid Governor." The *Los Angeles Times*, the *New York Times*, and national radio and television stations interviewed me. Media in Australia, New Zealand, and even China reported on the story. The reactions ranged from hysterical laughter—that a nurse could be so threatening to the governor—to outrage. My only "crime" was that I was wearing a nurse's uniform. The officers that detained me admitted to this. I never received a formal apology for this ridiculous treatment and violation of my civil rights. Some people equated it with Rosa Parks being asked to move to the back of the bus. The American Civil Liberties Union (ACLU) even reviewed my case.

What have I learned from all of this? Nurses must stand up for their patients and their profession no matter what. We have a voice, we are strong, and people will listen. We have power! I did not plan what happened to me, but I found myself in the position of having to take on the bigger-than-life governor of California, who had sky-high approval ratings when he took office, to protect my patients and the staffing ratios we nurses had fought so hard for. At times, it felt like David battling Goliath. But we nurses brought him down, just as David slew the giant; because we spoke out and persevered, the governor backed down. He stopped attacking the ratios and even chose a Democrat as his chief of staff. His poll numbers dropped to an all-time low. We won and saved our ratios. Most important, the patients in California hospitals won.

• • •

KELLY DiGIACOMO, RN, lives and works in Sacramento California, has practiced in the areas of cardiology, labor and delivery, and pediatrics for over twenty years, has served on the Board of Directors for the California Nurses Association and is a past Region President, and is currently completing her Master of Science in Nursing degree.

Saving the Carney

Penny Connolly

For over thirty years, I've worked as a nurse at Carney Hospital—a community hospital owned by the Caritas Christi Health Care system—in Dorchester, Massachusetts. The Carney provides critical services to a diverse community, including many patients with little or no income.

In October 2007, the Caritas system announced that they were going to close the hospital for financial reasons. The Massachusetts Nurses Association (MNA) asked the nurses who live in the area to meet to see what we could do to save the Carney. We spoke with the neighborhood health associations, clinics, and neighborhood groups. The consensus was that the hospital was viable and that the community couldn't afford to lose it. Other neighborhood health care groups in the community had been meeting to fight the closing, and they contacted us and suggested we all band together.

In March 2008, we joined with the neighborhood health association in Dorchester. Along with this group we met with the mayor, with other elected officials, and with members of the community to argue that closing the Carney would have a devastating impact on the community. At these meetings, we presented data on the patients served by the Carney and why closing the hospital would have a devastating impact on the community. We explained that the Carney treated many patients insured by Medicaid, who would have trouble getting care in in-town hospitals. Many patients treated at the Carney had psychiatric issues, and our adult psychiatric unit, geriatric-psych unit, and adolescent psychiatry unit were essential in the continuum of care for these patients in the community.

We also determined that the financial impact on the community if all the people who were employed by the hospital were out of a job would be significantly negative. Even though we have some complex patients, we were getting reimbursed at a lower price than many in-town hospitals. We made the case that we gave quality care at a lower price than those hospitals.

Finally, after seven long months, the new president of Caritas Christi announced in May 2008 that they would keep the hospital open.

Nurses like myself fought the closing because we knew how valuable the hospital is. Most of the nurses have been there for years. We know our patients—many of whom depend on the Carney for care for chronic conditions. We also know the people in the community. They're our neighbors, our friends, sometimes our coworkers. We were proud of our hospital and we could not let it close. We fought for it, and it stayed open.

• • •

PENNY CONNOLLY, RN, has worked at the Carney Hospital in Dorchester, Massachusetts, for over thirty years; she won the hospital's President Award which recognizes an employee for compassion, accountability, respect, and excellence in service.

Part 9
STILL FIGHTING

Some people didn't want me to include this section in this book. These are stories of defeats or of constant battling, not of victories. They are stories that highlight frustration, not success. In these stories, nurses fight to move the proverbial two steps forward only to be catapulted three steps back. In the typically sweet, sappy, and widely advertised motivational books that target nurses, "happy endings" are de rigueur.

Unfortunately, as nurses know better than most of us, real life (and death) tends to be messier than that. Indeed, as we have seen recently, many of the victories nurses thought they had secured after endless battles are now put into question whenever there is a budget crunch in academia, an assault by organized medicine, or cost-cutting in hospitals and other health care institutions.

I began writing about nursing during one of those periods. I entered on the scene during the nursing shortage of the 1980s, when hospitals and other facilities seemed finally to get it, and nurses were winning better benefits, more money, and more voice. Then came the restructuring of the 1990s, and all those hard-won victories were eroded. Nurses had to fight their being replaced by unskilled personnel and to maintain their wages and benefits. In hospitals, old ideas of team and functional nursing that had been abandoned in favor of primary nursing were once again resurrected. In home care, schools, and psychiatric facilities, nurses were once again put on the defensive. Then in the early 2000s everyone admitted that there was a nursing shortage, and suddenly it was "Quick, where are the nurses? We have to do something to get more nurses."

That lasted about five years, and now we are back to the future. In Canada, hospitals want to replace registered nurses with licensed practical nurses. In the United States, hospitals now insist there is no shortage of nurses. Why? Because patients are getting all the care they need? Hardly. It's because they are misallocating their resources and want to cut costs on the back of nursing care. The take-home message here is that the fight is never over.

That's why I think these stories belong right here, at the end of this volume. The stories in this final section don't have neat and tidy endings, and that's exactly why I included them. Patient advocacy doesn't only involve taking occasional risks; it means being ready to lose a battle or two along the way but still continue the struggle. It also involves winning and then discovering that winning isn't the end of the story.

Continuing to stand up and advocate is, after all, what great nurses have always done and why their profession has continued to advance. To me, the nurses whose narratives conclude this book offer no less inspiration than any of the others we've heard along the way. They view any setbacks or failures they've encountered as the midwife of further persistence. Such nurses deserve the last word in this collection because real progress is made only when some people continue to stand up for what's right, regardless of the odds against them and without any guarantee of success that (much to the surprise of everyone) may be right around the corner.

The Male Midwife

Gregg Trueman

About twenty years ago I was a twenty-eight-year-old nursing student starting his second career in a Catholic, hospital-based school of nursing program. Learning the medicine every nurse needs to know was a joyful and rigorous academic undertaking. I delighted in my growing understanding of the human body and the human condition, studying the nature of suffering, and learning how to nurse the experience of birth and death. This was to become my life's work, and I was hooked from the very beginning.

The problem was, just as I was entering nursing, women were beginning to assert themselves in the Second Wave of the feminist movement. Although I fully supported that movement, I was distressed to find that, in the name of feminism, women were insisting that a male midwife was a contradiction in terms.

Obstetrics nurses—all women—would ask me, "What could you possibly know about this thing called birth?" Sure, I had read everything I was assigned to read, and then some. My professor taught me about assessing and responding to the physiological stages connected to childbirth. She taught us about breathing and about the transitions in the family as a result of pregnancy and birth. My classmates and I had all studied the uncertainties between here and there . . . and *still*, what could *I* possibly know about giving birth? What was I to do?

And so, one day after classes ended and before the practicum began, I called my mother. Being the sage giver of life—four times over—she simply stated: "*Do not ever* argue with the mother! She knows what is happening with her; give her what she needs." Mom's words were prophetic, to be sure.

Early in my labor and delivery (L&D) practicum I was assigned to a young family about to welcome their first child into the world. It was at once a magical and tentative time for this petite and beautiful twenty-four-year-old mother-to-be and her handsome six-feet-four-inch partner. The family, my contemporaries, had longed for what was about to come true and we were all excited about baby soon to be born. Young mum's labor pains, however, overshadowed the enthusiasm they both shared for what was about to be made real. As it was, my presence and my studies in obstetrical nursing made me the midwife, responsible for their care and the delivery of their baby. I was their guide during a life-altering transition; I was a caring witness to the uncertainties inherent in child birth. All of this, and yet my sex—according to my experienced colleagues—kept me a "stranger."

Through the first eight hours of their labor, the three of us breathed together, laughed, and called on the past to make meaning of the present. In between the breathing and the laughing and the walking and the sobbing, we talked about parenthood and christened the child's future with all of the kind intentions and bountiful best wishes two parents naturally have for their unborn child. As my shift came to an end and it was time for me to think about leaving, young mum looked up and said, "Please don't go, I can't do this without you."

I asked my professor for permission to stay for an extra shift, much to the chagrin of the OB nurses on the unit. I told my teacher—a jubilant and joyful Jamaican midwife—that I had never felt as useful or as connected to any patient since I set sail on this journey called nursing. She agreed that my presence was meaningful and ran interference for me with the OB nurses sitting at the desk debating my suitability to serve.

Over the next eight hours, the young mother didn't progress much in her labor. At her urging, and even though baby's heart rate was strong and stable, I approached the obstetrical resident and asked for another assessment about her failure to progress.

My advocacy raised the ire of the experienced nurses at the desk—which I answered to later. Hearing this dissension among the nursing ranks didn't do much to bring comfort to an uncertain young family. By the time the resident physician attended the room, the fetal heart rate was decelerating and young mum was in distress, even though she was still only dilated to three centimeters. Minutes later she was headed to the surgical suite for an emergency caesarean section and I was caring for the young dad while he trembled in fear at the thought of losing both his beloved wife and his baby. Twenty-eight minutes later one of the neonatal nurses arrived and told dad that his wife was fine and had given birth to a healthy nine pound, ten ounce boy. The young dad was now a father, and his wife a much relieved mother.

Inspired by my experiences in labor and delivery, I reached out to the most prominent midwife in the province to declare my intention of becoming "an exceptional L&D nurse." I sought her advice on how I ought to plan the remainder of my nursing program. Enthusiastic and full of the possible, I spoke with "Doreen" and, upon hearing the baritone timbre of my voice, I was immediately put in my proper place. Without hesitation she replied: "You're a man; what could you possibly know about childbirth? . . . We [midwives] don't want you . . . we'll make it hard for you . . ."—and that was the end of that.

My nursing program was not yet complete, and so I soldiered on. This was not the first time my sex was held up as a defining characteristic of my developing practice. Over the next year and a half, my sense of possibility was again ignited by a palliative care home care nurse who remains to this day one of my many heroines. Anna taught me how to marry compassion and grace. She quietly showed me the swell of similarities in the transitions that usher life in and with which we make our final exit. Over a twelve-week practicum, my commitment to hospice palliative care was born and has flourished ever since.

Even though my intention to help patients gracefully navigate their final exit became a reality, I have always wondered why I could not serve as a midwife. Men's capacity to nurse, just like women's, is founded on an ability to work together, with our patients, with our colleagues, and with our communities. I chose to learn how to practice nursing, rather than medicine, because the tools that I wished to bring to work, in addition to my skill, knowledge, and experience, were care and compassion; I wanted to be connected to health as opposed to treating illness.

Since my undergraduate days, I have earned licensure and practice as a primary and end-of-life care nurse practitioner; I am working on my second PhD and teach in an undergraduate nursing program. My stories as an undergraduate and my experiences in practice now inform the manner in which I educate the many male *and female* nursing students on their own journey to becoming a professional nurse. It is not a coincidence that my guidance as a professor is similar to the counsel received by many female medical students in the 1960s: "Stay the course, study and work hard, and ignore the gossip from those who do not know your heart."

The twentieth century, when I went to nursing school, is history, and the twenty-first century is now well upon us. In the United States, the first African American sits in the Oval Office, and women around the globe are parliamentarians, prime ministers, and presidents of sovereign nations. Women are CEOs of health care systems and investment banks, and yet men in nursing schools still experience gender-based ridicule and professional marginalization daily as they seek their rightful role as a professional nurse.

One day, perhaps, the idea of a male midwife might be as normative as the thought of a female surgeon, or Justice of the Supreme Court, or Canadian Prime Minister, but not, regrettably, today.

• • •

GREGG TRUEMAN, NP, PhD, MN, CHPCN(c), is an Acute Care Nurse Practitioner (primary and hospice palliative care) for the Calgary Urban Project Society, an assistant professor in the Faculty of Health and Community Studies at Mount Royal University, and is preparing for his PhD candidacy examinations in the Faculty of Medicine at the University of Calgary.

Fighting for Our Vets

Edmond O'Leary

Between 1974 and 1986 I served in the U.S. Air Force Nurse Corps. I had the honor and privilege of serving with the men and women who made sacrifices to make our country great. After returning from the service, I began a long career as a nurse in the U.S. Department of Veterans Affairs (VA) where I have cared for prisoners of war (POWs) from Vietnam, Korea, and World War II. I met several distinguished members of the armed forces, such as General James Doolittle, Chappie James, and nurses from the Bataan Death March. I was on the team that received and helped repatriate the Iran hostages who were held captive for 444 days. Hearing their stories and learning how they have survived while coping with horrendous conditions and unbelievable pain, suffering, and torture made me honor these American heroes more. It made me proud to wear my uniform. Although I am proud of my uniform, sometimes I have not been proud of how our veterans and nurses are treated. When I've seen unsafe conditions, my commitment to honoring our soldiers' sacrifices means I know I have to do something to change these conditions.

This is why, one day when I was evening and night charge nurse of a surgical intensive care unit, I had to say No. I watched the care and quality of treatment become unacceptable and deplorable. Over a period of twelve months the mortality rate went from less than 3 percent to above 10 percent. I had to take action and seek justice for my nurses and the patients we served. These problems arose in great part because surgical residents—some of whom came from cultures where women were not considered equal to men—used this as an excuse to behave disrespectfully and unprofessionally to our nurses, who were mostly female. When a female nurse would call the resident to come to the unit because there were changes in the condition of the patient, for example, the physician would not respond in a timely manner because a woman—the nurse—had called him. When they did respond, they would fondle and touch the nurses in inappropriate ways.

I spoke to the physicians and told them that their actions were unacceptable and had best stop. They just laughed it off. I gathered my nurses into a conference and told them, "From today on, if any physician touches or fondles you, inform him the first time this is not acceptable to do. The next time he does it, slap him and yell for help."

The next day a physician who had already received a warning pushed his luck. He patted an RN's bottom. She slapped him and yelled for help. I called our security service and had him arrested for sexual abuse. He was carted off to jail. I called the chief of staff, who was a physician, and told him he needed to replace the on-call resident because he was now in jail and explained why. This got the attention of the other residents, but it was way too late for many of our patients. The hospital lost its accreditation to perform surgical procedures, and the program folded.

What this taught me and the other nurses I worked with is that you have to stand up. Standing up for ourselves is not just acting to protect ourselves. It's sometimes the only way we can act to protect our patients. In this case, the hospital closed. It didn't close because of our actions. It closed because it didn't deserve to stay open. By closing it, it allowed not only our nurses and many others to move on to better places and better jobs, it allowed our patients to be cared for in settings that provided truly high-quality care.

• • •

EDMOND O'LEARY, BSN, RN, is a nurse at the Durham Veterans Affairs Medical Center and president of UAN Local Number 1.

We Are the Experts

Karen Higgins

I've been a nurse for thirty-four years, and for a lot of those years nursing administration took care of us and made sure things were going well so that all I had to do was go in and take care of patients. But during the 1990s, things changed, and nurses like myself felt that nursing administration wasn't supporting bedside RNs but had become a part of the high-level hospital management team representing the financial and survival imperatives of hospitals. For the first time, I was convinced that if anyone was going to ensure patients were safe, it would have to be staff nurses. I first recognized this when the hospital began to lay off nurses and hire unlicensed people. Initially, administrators insisted that "they're coming in to help you; they're going to be your helping hands." But as I watched nurses leaving my hospital, the "helping hands" seemed to be pushing nurses out the door rather than helping RNs at the bedside.

My job became more difficult. I was now responsible not only for the patient but also for the unlicensed person replacing my former nurse colleague. Administrators told us this was okay because these aides were only doing routine "tasks." The problem is that nothing a nurse does is a routine task. We have to use our knowledge and experience to do every single thing we do. And any nurse with experience knows that there is really not much in the hospital that is routine. Everything can turn into a catastrophe in a second flat. I watched the restructuring of nursing out of the hospital and thought, "This is so wrong; it's so dangerous not only to the patient."

I was involved in the Massachusetts Nurses Association (MNA) and suggested that we needed to talk to nurses from all over the state to find out if they were experiencing what I and my colleagues were experiencing. We invited nurses to come and discuss these issues. What we discovered was that nursing layoffs and replacement of nurses with unlicensed personnel was indeed a huge problem throughout the state. The seeds of our Safe Care Campaign began at that meeting, in October 1994.

For the past twelve years we have been campaigning for a patient safety legislative agenda. This agenda included pushing bills on the state level to set safe patient limits for nurses; a bill to require the clear identification of licensed providers so that patients know who is a nurse and who isn't; a bill to provide whistleblower protection for nurses; and a bill to require hospitals to track staffing levels along with a variety of patient safety indicators, such as patient falls, bed-sores, hospital-acquired infection rates, and so on. The campaign has also involved an effort to reach out and talk to the media about these issues, and an effort to mobilize the non-nurse community, health care, and labor advocacy groups to join our effort to protect patients.

For me, the role I played in this fight came as a big surprise. I am not someone who feels comfortable standing up in public. Quite the contrary. I feel uncomfortable in the spotlight. But we decided to have a rally at the Massachusetts Statehouse in Boston in 1995, and I was approached and asked to speak. As for many others, getting up in public and speaking is one of my biggest nightmares. My first instinct was to say no, absolutely not. Get somebody else. But then I said to myself, "If you truly believe that we need to make a stand on this issue, then you have to stop and do what you're asked to do. If they ask you to speak, you need to speak." I said yes.

That's how I found myself on the steps of the Statehouse with about 150 nurses standing in front of me. There were also dozens of newspaper, television, and radio reporters there. This was the first time anybody had stepped forward to say publicly that hospitals in Massachusetts weren't safe. Although I knew hospital administrators—including some of my own—would be watching and wouldn't like what I had to say, that wasn't my primary worry. I didn't care whether the hospital liked it or not because it was a reality. But I felt uneasy about my qualifications to speak: "Who am I," I thought, "to say things are wrong here?" Up until that point I had always felt, "I'm just a staff nurse. What I do is take care of patients—or I try to take care of patients." It was terrifying because I thought, "Who am I to stand up in front of a group of people and do this?"

Now I realize that we, as staff nurses, are the backbone of health care. We are what keeps health care running. Now I tell every nurse I meet, You are the experts. As far as taking care of patients, you are the experts in whatever nursing field you are in—whether it's medical-surgical, oncology, or orthopedics. You need to stand up and make it clear you are the experts. You are the direct connection to the patient. Before, the mantra was, We are just staff nurses, and nursing administration will take care of us because we cannot understand the bigger picture. What I realized in that terrifying moment on the Statehouse steps before I opened my mouth to speak was that this mantra was no longer true—if it ever was. We are the experts, and we need to step up to the plate.

• • •

KAREN HIGGINS, RN, is a critical care nurse and is a past President of the Massachusetts Nurses Association and the Co-Chair of the Coalition to Protect Massachusetts Patients.

A Collective Voice

Diane Sosne

My maternal grandmother was a survivor of New York City's historic Triangle Shirtwaist Fire in which 146 factory workers, mostly young immigrant women, died in the fire or jumped to their deaths. This tragedy spurred legislation for improved factory safety standards and the growth of the International Ladies' Garment Workers' Union.

When choosing my career path, little did I know how my grandmother's history would affect me. Thirty-eight years ago, I became a registered nurse. In nursing school I was taught that the basis for good patient care was nursing care plans. As a psychiatric nurse I dutifully wrote lots of care plans. While nursing care plans are needed to help individual patients improve, I quickly noticed there were still gaps in the care patients received.

Drawing on the tragedy my grandmother survived, I was inspired to fix these gaps using the collective voice of nurses fighting for quality patient care for all.

Collective action has helped address one of the most serious problems that nurses and patients face today—the erosion of patient care due to hospital short-staffing. From the start of our local nurses' union in Seattle, our hospital nurse members, as well as nurses wanting to join with us, recited story after story of how they felt they had to compromise the care they gave patients due to short-staffing. One particularly poignant story was a nurse recounting how she did not have the time to provide comfort to a dying patient. She went home that night in tears, knowing she was not able to provide the care that was needed.

After listening to hundreds of similar painful admissions by staff nurses, we decided we needed to take bigger collective action and turned to our national union to create an SEIU National Nurse Survey. This survey of ten thousand nurses documented the harm to patients from short-staffing in 1993. The results of this survey were alarming enough that Congress commissioned the Institute of Medicine (IOM) of the National Academy of Science to study nurse staffing levels in hospitals and nursing homes and to determine what effect those levels had on quality of care. The IOM report, "Nursing Staff in Hospitals and Nursing Homes: Is It Adequate?" released to Congress in 1996, said the committee was shocked at the lack of available data linking nurse staffing levels with quality of care in hospitals and called for a national research investigation of hospital practices related to quality of patient care.

Unfortunately, this national focus has not yet led to a fix, but it did shine a spotlight on this problem. As a result we have pending national nurse staffing legislation to provide an industry-wide solution. And we also have legislation in one state (California) that guarantees safe nurse-to-patient ratios.

All patients deserve safe staffing. Some of the patients who deserve safe staffing are now nurses themselves, and, as nurses age, there will be an increasing number of nurses in the patient role. I was recently one of them after breaking my ankle in the Philippines and being raced back to Seattle for ankle surgery. I was so grateful to the nurses who took great care of me in both countries.

As many of us baby boomer nurses get ready to leave the nursing profession, thousands of care plans later, we can look back on our careers as having left an indelible mark of activism and collectivism. As union nurses, we not only stood up for the patients in our care but stood together to strengthen our profession and improve staffing. The groundwork for health care reform and quality care to benefit all patients is well on its way. As I grow older and anticipate being a patient again someday, I will still be fighting for patient care, and I hope younger nurses will fight for me and all those patients who depend on their collective advocacy.

· · ·

DIANE SOSNE, RN, MN, President of SEIU Healthcare 1199NW, Seattle, was previously a psychiatric nurse at Group Health Cooperative in Seattle and is currently a member of the SEIU Nurse Alliance and also sits on the International Executive Board for the Service Employees International Union (SEIU).

We Will Not Be Silenced

Carol Youngson

The saga began in 1993 and led to the longest medical inquest in Canadian history. I was then the nurse in charge of the Pediatric Cardiac Operating Room at the Health Sciences Center in Winnipeg, Manitoba, a position I had held for several years. In June, our cardiac surgeon, Dr. Kim Duncan, left to practice in the United States. In mid-February 1994, Dr. Jonah Odim arrived to take his place. The Pediatric Cardiac team, including myself, was pleased we had been able to attract a physician with such shining credentials: Ivy League education, years of specialty training, and, perhaps most impressive, experience working at the Boston Children's Hospital, a world-renowned center for pediatric cardiac surgery. The team expectation was that, as Dr. Odim and our group learned to work together, we would gradually restart the program, beginning with low-risk cases and progressing to more difficult ones.

Over the following months, we became painfully aware that impressive credentials on paper don't necessarily translate into competent, let alone stellar, performances in the operating room (OR). Almost immediately we began to see technical problems—for example, repairs failing and having to be redone, excessive bleeding of patients on the operating table, and unnecessarily long heart-pump runs. Cases we had always considered routine were turning into nightmares. If the children did survive surgery, they were being left with severe and life-threatening complications.

The first child, Gary Caribou, died one month after Dr. Odim started work. Within the next month, three other children, Jessica Ulimaumi, Vinay Goyal, and Daniel Terziski died. Gary, Jessica, and Vinay had undergone ventricular septal defect repairs performed by Dr. Odim. This type of surgery is considered low to medium risk and had been routine for us. All three of those children bled to death. Of

240

course, our prior surgeon had lost some patients. All surgeons do. But he rarely lost them because they bled to death.

The second child, nine-month old Jessica Ulimaumi, was sent after surgery to the pediatric intensive care unit (PICU) on an extracorporeal membrane oxygenatator (ECMO) machine, which is a form of bypass used as a last-ditch attempt to support a patient unable to maintain adequate blood pressure and oxygenation. Three days later, Dr. Odim decided to remove Jessica from the ECMO machine without any OR staff being present. Had they been present, they would have had the sutures, clamps, and other instruments he needed. Supposedly, this was how it had been done in Boston, but it certainly wasn't our mode of operation.

The result of his Lone Ranger actions was a catastrophe. While removing small tubes from Jessica's heart, a piece of tubing was not clamped, and she bled out through it onto the bed. During this bedside procedure, the site on the right atrial chamber of the heart where tubes had been inserted was torn so Dr. Odim had to clamp off this hole in Jessica's tiny heart with his fingers because there were no surgical instruments or OR staff at the bedside. Jessica's parents were not told of this at the time of her death and only at the inquest did they learn why their daughter had died. There was nothing in the surgical notes, progress notes, or anywhere else in the chart to indicate that this event had taken place.

We pediatric cardiac nurses told our nursing supervisors what was happening. They took our concerns seriously; however, the department heads to whom they passed on these concerns did not. Nothing happened. Over and over again, the same thing happened. We complained to nursing supervisors. They relayed our concerns and were ignored. I became so concerned that I began to make notes on my home computer about some of the incidents. This record proved to be invaluable later.

The fifth death, that of Alyssa Still, occurred on May 6, 1994. By that time, Dr. Odim had done eleven open-heart procedures on ten patients—with an alarming 50 percent mortality rate. And finally, the cardiac anesthetists, who shared the nurses' concerns, threatened to withdraw their services. In response, a committee known as the

Wiseman Committee, after its chair Dr. Nathan Wiseman, was established to review the pediatric cardiac program. I was the *only nurse* among several doctors on the committee. Over the next few months, we reviewed the cases but at no time were the real issues—in particular, surgical competence, lack of communication, and speed of program development—addressed. Interestingly, none of Dr. Wiseman's notes mentioned the nursing concerns discussed at the meetings.

Over the summer of 1994, the Pediatric Cardiac Team did only low-risk cases with mainly good outcomes, except for Shalynn Piller and Aric Baumann, who both died in August. We continued to see technical problems in the OR and some near-fatal mishaps. Under pressure from Dr. Giddins, the cardiologist, and Dr. Odim, the cardiac surgeon, we embarked on a full program September 7, 1994, which meant we would accept all patients. No one, especially the nursing staff, felt we were ready for that. Unfortunately, we had no say in the matter. One week later, Marietess Capili died, followed by Erica Bichel on October 4, and Ashton Feakes on November 11. Again, we nurses repeatedly went through the proper channels to report our concerns about Dr. Odim's competence. And once again, it seemed that no one was prepared to do anything about the situation. We tried to decide what the best course of action would be. Should we talk to the parents? To the media? Where could we go to be heard?

Personally, I could no longer walk into the waiting room, take a child out of his or her parents' arms, and go into the OR. I assigned that job to other nurses who didn't do cardiac cases on a daily basis. I wanted to tell those parents to take their child and run!

On November 27, 1994, my worst nightmare came true. For almost a year, I had watched Dr. Odim struggle with the cannulation (insertion of tubes) into tiny blood vessels, often tearing them in the process. I was sure that this would eventually result in the death of a child in the OR, and on this day I saw it happen. The repair of Jesse Maguire's heart was complete, and things were looking pretty hopeful for this tiny three-day-old. As I turned for an instant toward the instrument table beside me, I heard a gasp.

When I looked back at Jesse's heart, I saw that the aortic cannula, which supplies oxygenated blood to the child from the bypass machine, had been knocked out! In trying to reinsert the cannula,

Dr. Odim tore and destroyed the aortic repair he had just completed. The repair was only millimeters from the cannula site. He now had to redo everything. This meant more bypass time for an infant too small to tolerate such a lengthy procedure. Jesse died on the operating table after thirteen hours of surgery.

This time I went straight to Dr. Brian Postl, then the head of Pediatrics. He promised me he would look into the situation. It was not, however, until another neonate, Erin Petkau, died on December 21, 1994, following routine, low-risk surgery that something was done: The program was shut down and Dr. Odim encouraged to take a "vacation." By then twelve children were dead. A cardiac surgeon and a cardiac anesthetist from Toronto's Hospital for Sick Children conducted an external review of the program and found numerous problems.

On February 14, 1995, the Health Sciences Center issued a press release stating that the pediatric cardiac program was under review for six months because the patient outcomes had not achieved the hoped-for standards. Parents of the deceased children began to demand answers. Why weren't they told about the problems? Why weren't they told that this was Dr. Odim's first job? Why weren't they told about the review done by the Wiseman Committee in the summer of 1994? And perhaps most important, why weren't they given the option to take their children elsewhere, especially those children requiring complex, high-risk surgery?

These questions plus many others formed the basis for the Pediatric Cardiac Inquest, headed by Provincial Court Judge Murray Sinclair, which ran from March 1995 until October 1998. (Note: Inquests find fact, not fault.) For five days during that six-week period, I was under cross-examination by the surgeon's lawyer. I was also cross-examined by lawyers for the anesthetists, the Health Sciences Center, and the families. Parents, grandparents, and other members of the deceased patients' families sat in the gallery while I testified. Sometimes I could see or hear them weeping as I related the events I had witnessed concerning their child. It was very difficult for me to talk about the details of a child's death knowing the parents were present.

In fall 1995, the Health Sciences Center decided that the evidence provided by the nursing staff could prove to be a *conflict of interest* for the Center. We nurses were advised by the Center that we should seek our own legal counsel. In other words, our employer had set us adrift. We were unable to secure legal counsel from the Canadian Nurses Protection Society because we were not being sued. Desperate and terrified, we approached the Manitoba Association of Registered Nurses (MARN) for help. Isobel Boyle, the director of patient services at Children's Hospital, set up a meeting with MARN.

Diana Davidson-Dick, then the executive director of MARN, listened to our story and took our concerns to their board of directors. Our situation seemed all too familiar to Diana, and she appreciated that we nurses needed our own separate legal standing. The MARN hired lawyers to represent us and paid for our legal expenses. Diana sat in that courtroom while several of us testified, a visible reminder that MARN was behind us. I feel strongly that if we had been forced to depend on the Health Sciences Center to act on our behalf we might be in a very different situation today. As well, we will always feel gratitude to Colleen Suche of the law firm Suche-Gange. There were days when I thought I couldn't go into that courtroom again, but Colleen was there with us throughout the whole ordeal. She never backed down, always standing up for us personally and for our profession.

The Pediatric Cardiac Inquest lasted for three and a half years with 278 days of testimony, 86 witnesses, and almost 50,000 pages of recorded evidence. It is the first inquest in Canadian history where registered nurses had separate legal standing. At the conclusion of the inquest, all parties were asked to submit their own recommendations to Judge Sinclair. Highlights of the lengthy document submitted by nurses included:

1. Patients and families must be recognized as members of the decision-making team; that is, informed consent cannot occur unless *all the information* is shared. Marietess Capili's father put it so well when he said, "My right to serve my child's best interest was stolen from me by lies and misrepresentation."

2. Nurses must be equal partners with physicians in health care. This would help ensure responsible nursing as well as recognition of the importance of nursing.

3. All participants in the health care system should be held accountable consistent with their authority, power, and degree of control. Currently, nurses are accountable and liable, but without the requisite authority, power, or influence.

4. Reporting lines must be logical and well known within the facility.

While this story had a tragic ending for far too many young infants, children, and their families, the inquest did vindicate our efforts to advocate for our patients. We stood up and would not stand down, and Justice Sinclair's final comments took the hospital to task for its failure to act on our concerns. In his report, Judge Sinclair found that eight of the twelve deaths were preventable, three might have been prevented, and one was not preventable. The report ended: "It is clear that legitimate warnings and concerns raised by nurses were not always treated with the same respect or seriousness as those raised by doctors. While there are many reasons for this, the attempted silencing of members of the nursing profession, and the failure to accept the legitimacy of their concerns meant that serious problems in the pediatric cardiac surgery program were not recognized or addressed in a timely manner. As a result, patient care was compromised."

I have since left bedside practice, but I have not stopped talking about nurses' need to stand up and speak about risks to patient care. This could happen to any nurse, anywhere. The only way to prevent this kind of event from happening again is for every nurse to speak out, despite personal and professional risk, when we see anything that jeopardizes our patients.

· · ·

CAROL YOUNGSON, RN, is a Registered Nurse with over forty years of experience, primarily in the Operating Room. In 1998, she left the nursing profession and currently works as a Medical Examiner Investigator for the Chief Medical Examiner in Manitoba, Canada. This story is adapted from a speech given by Carol Youngson.

Standing By One Patient

Faith Simon

One of the things I do as a nurse practitioner practicing pediatric and adolescent medicine in a rural health clinic in northern California—in a county with the fishing and logging industry in decline and thus a lot of poor people—is try to get people appropriate health care. This isn't always easy and demands persistence, patience, and sticking with the patient no matter what.

About a year ago, a sixteen-year-old whom I'd known for about eight years came into the office complaining that he didn't feel well. He hadn't felt well in a long time, he told me. And that was about it.

I asked him question after question, but all he would say was, "I don't feel well. My stomach hurts. My head hurts." He told me he hadn't eaten in a long time, and I could see that he'd lost a lot of weight and appeared depressed and agitated. He'd had some trouble in school in the past and I'd helped with that, so I'd known him as a troubled kid but not, as he was presenting now, as a sick kid.

I listened to his heart and lungs, I palpated and percussed his abdomen, I checked blood work, I asked him to journal his signs and symptoms looking for triggers, and still no medical diagnosis. I did tests to try to determine what was wrong with him, and test after test came back negative. As we talked, he confessed that he was using a lot of marijuana to deal with his problems and he'd feel worse when he was imminently out of pot. He would get agitated, out of control, and even hysterical. There didn't seem to be any physical cause of his problems. Which only made him more agitated and anxious. It became clear his problems were psychological.

As time progressed, the pot smoking became more of a problem and less of a help. It actually started producing more of the kinds of symptoms he was using it to temper. He was no longer going to school, and he was calling his mother at work every hour telling her that he wasn't feeling well and begging her to come home and help him.

246

I needed to get him mental health services. He had state-sponsored medical insurance that covered psychiatric care, but access was a barrier. Where we live, there are few mental health services available. The only child psychiatrist is one and a half hours away. Accessing mental health services is like a mission impossible.

This was not news to me. Because of the lack of services in our area, I'm forced to do a lot of mental health medicine. I have a few tools I use to assess someone's degree of depression and anxiety, and my workup on Paul suggested he was suffering from anxiety and depressive disorders. Because of lack of services, I am also forced to prescribe medications that should really be prescribed by a psychiatrist. Again, this situation is typical for nurses in rural medicine. We are forced to provide services our patients can't otherwise access. But it's very tricky prescribing medications that you do not have expertise in—particularly with children and adolescents—and there are more and more black box alerts on drugs warning of suicide and other potentially dangerous or fatal complications. So, like many of my colleagues practicing in rural areas, I felt on shaky ground. I preferred he see a psychiatrist who really knows about these medications.

So I set about trying to find a psychiatrist for Paul and encountered obstacle after obstacle. Paul was rejected from one program because he was sixteen not fifteen. Then he was rejected from another because he was sixteen and not eighteen. To become a (county) mental health patient, Paul and one of his parents had to see an "evaluator" for three or more hour-long sessions who in turn might or might not refer to a therapist who might or might not refer to a psychiatrist.

Unfortunately, these "evaluators" are not licensed therapists or counselors. They are minimally trained crisis workers used as gatekeepers. Each time Paul and a parent met with an "evaluator," they would become distressed. Even if the session went well, the person would often not call back for weeks. Time after time, Paul and his family would meet mental health technicians or assistants who would upset him and/or his parents. He had yet to meet with the therapist (who would maybe—that's maybe—agree to pass him on to a psychiatrist).

In the meantime, someone had to help Paul deal with his increasingly serious problems. By now Paul was having daily and sometimes hourly panic attacks, punching holes in the walls of his bedroom, making escalating demands and threats toward his family. I remained the only "professional" involved in his care.

My best option seemed to be pharmaceutical, so I was prescribing drugs that were complex and that I was not completely comfortable with. I was trying to change doses, mixes, trying to calm him down. I was also trying to do therapy, which I am not trained to do, so that he could move beyond saying "I don't feel well" and verbalize what was really troubling him. I tried to set up some exercise programs for him. I tried to get him interested in doing something at home so that he would do more than sit around doing nothing except calling his mother every hour at work.

Our goal was to make the hour and a half drive over this terribly windy road to reach the only child psychiatrist in the county. It proved as difficult as making a journey across the ocean. As I grew more uncomfortable prescribing medications for Paul, I finally said, "no more" and referred him to a pediatrician. But the pediatrician had even less training in mental health than I did and simply lost patience with Paul. I could sit in a room with Paul, and he would blow up at me and I could tolerate it, but the pediatrician couldn't.

By now, Paul was becoming increasing violent, suicidal, and more and more distrustful of a system that seemed to refuse to help him. So I got an adult psychiatrist involved. He finally took over medication prescription and management. But he did no therapy and was difficult for the family to reach with questions or even for prescription renewals. He saw Paul only every eight weeks—not to do therapy but only to review the meds.

It was hardly surprising when Paul got even worse. He began to threaten his mother. She called the police, and he was taken to the nearby local emergency room (ER). I hoped this would pave the way for Paul to get a real psychiatric workup, a better medication regimen, and some stability in his care. But not in our system. Each time the cops came, they took him to the ER, he would be seen by a mental health worker—not a licensed therapist or psychiatrist—who, because Paul had calmed down by then, would decree that he was not an "imminent threat" to himself and others. So he wasn't sent to a psychiatric facility to be evaluated and perhaps stabilized. For that to happen, apparently, he would have had to have a proverbial gun pointing at his head with the trigger cocked.

Five times he was sent to the ER. Five times a crisis worker insisted that he wasn't a real threat. Five times he came home.

The only advance we made was to get him into a transitional youth program that was supposed to help him get a job so that at least he would have some structure in his life. But even here, we encountered the same old obstacle course. One program deemed him ineligible because he was too young, another because he was too old. As we were searching for programs, the mental health system decided that if he didn't deal with his marijuana addiction no one could do anything for him. He was labeled noncompliant and uncooperative. So the transitional program refused to admit him before he got off the pot.

Of course, it was true, he did have a substance abuse problem, but underlying this was a serious psychological illness. Except no one wanted to help him with that illness so he could get off the pot, and no one would help him get off the pot so he could deal with the illness. He was directed to a completely different county agency that would ostensibly help him recover from his pot addiction so that he could get to the child psychiatrist. Unfortunately, there is no program in northern California that deals with withdrawal from marijuana. Why? Because no one considers marijuana to be a substance that produces problems with withdrawal.

Paul went into limbo for months. Since this was written, Paul has had many more ER presentations; two resulted in seventy-two-hour involuntary holds that sent him to two different psychiatric facilities from which he was discharged home to the nebulous local mental health services. Finally, he was arrested twice actually for assaulting his mom and spent three months in juvenile detention. When he turned eighteen, he was released to the transitional-age youth program and set up with housing, a job, and enrolled in community college. His psychiatric needs remain addressed only chemically, on four different medications, which he began to wean himself off of almost immediately. Most recently he quit school, quit his job, began having panic attacks again, and once again called desperately begging for help because he didn't feel good.

And I'm still with him. I'll be with him at least until he's in his twenties. I'm one of the only people he doesn't hate. I'm the only link with the health care system that he still trusts. But I can't remake the health care system all by myself. Even though I sure wish I could.

· · ·

FAITH SIMON, RN, FNP, is a family nurse practitioner who works in a rural clinic in Northern California. She was an emergency nurse for twenty years before becoming an FNP.